P9-DEA-035

Living Through Pain

Living Through Pain

Psalms and the Search for Wholeness

Kristin M. Swenson

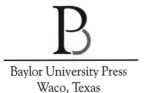

Baylor University Press
Waco, Texas

Book Design by Diane Smith
Cover Design by Bob Bubnis
Cover painting is *Pear Tree in Flowers* by Vincent Van Gogh, 1888 (Oil
on canvas, 73 cm x 46 cm; located in the Van Gogh Museum,
Amsterdam, The Netherlands).
Photo credit: Snark / Art Resource, NY

Library of Congress Cataloging-in-Publication Data

Swenson, Kristin M.
  Living through pain : Psalms and the search for wholeness / Kristin
M. Swenson.
      p. cm.
  Includes bibliographical references and index.
  ISBN 1-932792-15-5 (hardcover : alk. paper)
  1. Bible. O.T. Psalms--Criticism, interpretation, etc. 2. Pain--
Religious aspects--Christianity. 3. Suffering--Religious aspects--
Christianity. I. Bible. O.T. Psalms. English. Swenson. Selections.
2005. II. Title.

  BS1430.S82S94 2005
  248.8'6--dc22

                              2005012757

To my parents
L. Cecile Swenson and Richard E. Swenson

Contents

Acknowledgments

The word "wholism" today frequently refers to the integration of body, mind, and spirit. Seldom do we note how a person's social context and immediate community shape and are shaped by that person. The project of writing this book has been a humbling reminder that how and who I am is intimately connected to those who came before me, who are around me, and who will succeed me. I am grateful to my teachers; I owe a great debt to family, friends, and colleagues who have encouraged and supported me in this project; and I hope that with this project I extend something useful to others.

When I first began thinking about the topic, "biblical perspectives on pain," Patty Worley invited me to teach such a course for the Commonwealth Society, Virginia Commonwealth University's "institute for lifelong learning." I was a student in that class as much as anyone else, learning from the insights and experiences of a truly wonderful group of adults. Brian Cassel, John Quillin, and Mark Wood invited me to try out the topic in VCU's "Faith and the Life Sciences" course. The students in each of the courses that I teach never fail to challenge and enrich me in ways that are inestimably valuable.

The terms *family*, *friends*, and *colleagues* are artificially distinct in many cases. Members of my family have provided professional insights and critical ideas; friends have embraced me with loving support and encouragement; and I eat, bicker, and laugh with my colleagues. My mother and father, to whom this book is dedicated, have supported me in all ways. My sisters and their families have provided encouragement along the way.

I have benefited from many wonderful conversation partners, willing to share not only ideas but also the experiences that shaped them. Among them, I am especially grateful to Tom and Mary Boman, Charles Demm, Cliff Edwards, Rebecca Elstrom, Kathleen Gacek, Brad Graff, Denise Honeycutt, Doug Hoffman, Gina Kovarsky, David Kympton, Mindy Loiselle, Esther Nelson, Jen Pearson, Dan Perdue, Matt Sanford, Jack Spiro, Don Tubesing, Pat Watkins, Jon Waybright, Lynda Weaver-Williams, and Mark Wood. Their stories, questions, and keen insights give texture to this book. Some generously read rough chapters and offered suggestions for improvement. Faculty in VCU's School of World Studies by presence and model have cheered and inspired me to work when it seemed there was no end to the project. Library staff at VCU cheerfully processed interlibrary loan requests and the volumes that I borrowed.

Several people from VCU's medical center spent time talking to me about their experiences as physicians, nurses, and psychologists. They include David Cifu, Patrick Coyne, David Drake, Jeffrey Ericksen, David Hess, William McKinley, Thomas Mulligan, Thomas Smith, and William Walker. With considerable interest, passion, humor, and candor, they generously shared not only information but also thoughtful insights and wonder, and in so doing helped shape this book.

Carey Newman made this book happen. He has shepherded my fuzzy and wide-ranging ideas over mountains and through valleys, whistling all the way. I could not have asked for a better editor and companion in this project. I am grateful to Diane Smith and the staff at Baylor University Press for their work on this manuscript. Any mistakes that remain are my own.

Thanks to VCU's School of World Studies and College of Humanities and Sciences for granting me a semester research leave to aid in completing this book.

Introduction

"It's not such a wide gulf to cross, then, from survival to poetry." —Barbara Kingsolver

Telling politely curious people that you are working on a project concerning pain can be like pulling the plug on a cozy bath. Soon you sit there, naked and shivering, in an empty tub. Pain is hardly an inviting topic; yet I have found that once people get beyond an initial aversion, everybody has something to say about pain, frequently personal, and usually including wonder at the difficulty of pinning it down. Adding religion to the conversation stimulates the same paradoxical effects of aversion and fascination. I do not look like someone who is suffering chronic pain, so when people ask me what is the book that I have been working on, their first reaction to my answer frequently is a delayed "what?" After clarifying that the book concerns pain, "p-a-i-n," most people ask if it is about "physical pain" or about "pain in general, like psychological or emotional pain." My response to this question normally also addresses some part of the next question: Why the Psalms? In this introduction to *Living through Pain*, I anticipate that readers share the same kinds of questions, but also come to the book out of their own experiences wrestling with pain.

1

Consequently, I will briefly speak to those questions here and describe how the chapters that follow address aspects of the experience of pain in its multifaceted, ever-changing nature. However, because the topic of this book concerns two things about which people have a great number of opinions and considerable passion, I begin by telling what the book is not, in an effort to be fair to readers whose assumptions may not immediately be satisfied. If you are such a reader, I hope that you will suspend judgment long enough to read further. In the end, I hope that this book will prove useful to those who may be in pain and/or caring for persons in pain, and interesting to those curious about biblical perspectives on pain. Indeed, I hope that the experience of reading this book will be more like stepping into a steaming hot tub full of interesting people, easing aches and promising thought-provoking and engaging conversation.

In the face of questions about the relationship of religion to human suffering, or the role that pain plays in any given human life, it seems easiest to note first what this book is not. It is no more a sermon declaring how the Bible cures pain than it is a medical treatise proposing a particular course of treatment to render pain a thing of the past. This book is not an attempt to apply texts considered by many to be "Word of God" to the problem of pain as a kind of magic cure. Neither does it represent an effort to exonerate God and by whatever means, tell God's purpose for such an experience. I do not attempt to find a silver lining for pain or otherwise determine final effects or benefits. Pain is incredibly complicated and its management at least equally so. Some people want the pain that they have. Some of these people know that such is the case, and some only become aware that they want their pain when invited to see it with new eyes. *Living through Pain* is concerned with unwelcome pain and the efforts to mitigate or manage it.

I take as my starting point physical pain. However, I am especially concerned with chronic pain. I write "however" because pain that defies attempts to eliminate it and so is sustained for a period of time affects all aspects of a person — mind, spirit, and community, as well as body.[1] Indeed, for many people, the so-called mental or psychological distress of their condition is more painful than any physical aspect of it. Although I began this project primarily interested in what biblical texts have to say to and about physical pain, I have come to appreciate more deeply the inseparability of what we might call physical, emotional, psychological, and spiritual pain. Furthermore, social and cultural contexts also bear immediately on the experience of pain; and pain affects one's relationships to other people. This "whole person" nature of pain may be its most defining characteristic. It also makes discussing pain particularly challenging. Any candid discussion of pain is bound to come unbound. Digressions and turnabouts in discourse concerning pain are the norm and reflect the non-linear direction and polymorphous shape of the experience of pain itself. Pain is a personal thing, different for each individual, as unique as each one of us. Furthermore, the experience of pain is constantly changing for each person. This uniqueness and dynamism not only attests to the whole person nature of pain but also precludes precisely and finally identifying it with (any part of) the body, mind, spirit, or social relationships. Consequently, whatever we say about chronic pain is immediately relevant to experiences of social rejection, the loss of someone dear to us, unrequited love, professional failure; indeed any of the countless forms of suffering that we all experience in the course of our human lives. Finally, pain is difficult to describe, but you know it when you encounter it.[2]

The distinction between suffering and pain is more subtle, then, than simply identifying the former as an emotional or psychological experience and the latter as physical. Pain that does not go away affects a person's outlook, sense of self, spirituality, and relationship toward others. In dealing with pain, I am indeed concerned with a physical event; but it is also inseparable from all aspects of a person. As it negatively affects a person, it is appropriate to talk about "suffering pain." Similarly, chronic *suffering* affects all aspects of a person—physical as well as spiritual, emotional, psychological, and social—in ways that we are just beginning to understand. Emotionally traumatic experiences may instigate physical illness; and we speak of "painful suffering" in life events such as grief and loss.

As I note in the first chapter, there is a sobering rise in complaints of intractable pain, especially in the "industrialized West," and particularly in the United States. This may be because more people report it than they did before, it may be due to changes in lifestyle or perspective, or it may be the product of a combination of things. Whatever the case, despite increasing pharmacological treatments and medical technology, debilitating pain has gotten out of hand, and it is inseparable from great suffering. Pain has the capacity to fracture a person, creating gaps between body, mind, and spirit, as well as between the sufferer and others. That is, it creates distance between the sufferer and his or her life, preventing full participation in the promises, demands, challenges, and potential of any given moment as it happens. Pain preoccupies, prohibiting full engagement in the present, the only time any one of us really has. The quest to live *through* pain is the quest to reintegrate the fractured self into a whole person, fully alive at any given moment, even when that moment includes pain. It is, in a sense then, to take the suffering out of pain. To determine one's integrity, even in the presence of pain, is to make oneself whole, holy, and to heal. The process of identifying one's authentic self, in the present moment, wholly cognizant of and engaged in whatever bears on that experience, enables a person to find purpose and place; and sometimes the pain is mitigated, too.

I ask how psalms might aid in that process of reintegration and engagement for several reasons.[3] One is that I am trained as a biblical scholar, particularly of the Old Testament or "Hebrew Bible." But such training is inseparable from my abiding interest in these ancient texts, an interest that has flowered into an awe-filled respect for those involved in the centuries-long process of composing, editing, and compiling what we now have as "Bible." Another reason for listening to psalmic voices in considering the shades of pain is that they do not so easily divide a person into body, mind, and spirit. Neither do they separate an individual's experience from his or her social relationships. In other words, each of the psalms begins with the assumption that any person is a complicated product of internal and external relations. The six psalms that I have chosen to consider closely in light of the matter of pain speak out of both broken and reintegrating conditions, decrying pain's propensity to fracture, and seeking a means of being whole and engaged in life, even in light — or darkness — of great pain.

The candor with which the psalmists speak is an equally valuable characteristic of the psalms concerning the experience of pain. The psalms do not proffer a systematic theology; neither do they identify a diagnosis, prognosis, and course of treatment. Instead, they demonstrate the very real experience of persons wrestling with different aspects of the experience of pain. They offer a vocabulary and grammar for understanding and expressing aspects of that experience. Reading them as we do here is to discover that what may seem to be unbearably unprecedented suffering actually has company and sympathy in a shared human condition. Listening to these ancient poems may round off the cruel edge of loneliness that pain can bring.

Furthermore, they are considered religious texts—an obvious fact, yes, but remarkable for its implications. In their candor, these psalms do not mince words, and the result may be offensive to some religiously sensible readers. The psalmists complain, question, and express both great anger and a sense of betrayal at God as well as other people. The psalmists challenge a too easy theology that cannot abide the fact that bad things happen to good people and is scandalized by the questions and responses that such a fact elicits.[4] The psalmists do not deny, downplay, or dismiss honest reactions to the problem of pain. They tell them, wrestle with them in conversation with God and others, and they move through them. That the psalmists do not pontificate on answers to the problem of pain, but rather move through aspects of the experience, dignifies the process itself. That the psalmists' difficult words are canonized in sacred texts suggests that such dynamic wrestling has a place, even in a "godly" life.

Finally, yet another reason to consider the psalms in thinking about pain is that they are a part of our cultural atmosphere and landscape.[5] The Bible is indisputably influential, regardless of one's religious faith or lack thereof. Even as it is misunderstood and misused, the Bible permeates the cultural atmosphere of much of the world. Psalms, especially among the books of the Bible, exert a powerful influence, representing more than any other biblical book varied and heartfelt responses to a wide range of human experiences. We do well, then, to examine the psalms for their contribution to the ways in which we understand and seek to manage pain, even when we disagree with or otherwise differ from them.

I include a translation of the psalms for the readers' convenience. There are more than twenty English translations of the Bible, reflecting the diversity of its audience. The translations from the original Hebrew that I include here, and on which I base my discussion, are my own. All translation is interpretation. I hope that I have rendered these texts as true to their meaning and sense as is possible for our purposes here, retaining enough of what is foreign to remind us of the texts' antiquity and so to temper our arrogant inclination to read them as if they were written in twenty-first century English, while rendering them familiar enough to accept their invitation of engagement.

The texts are rooted in faith, coming to us through the hands of those who believed in the God of and to whom they speak. Consequently, in the chapter discussions of individual psalms, I have rendered the words transliterated *Elohim, YHWH,* and *Adonai* as "God" in the context of discussion for the sake of simplicity, noting the distinction of terminology where it enriches the chapter's investigation. However, I retain the distinctions in my translation of the psalms, where I translate them "God," "YHWH," and "Lord," respectively. Like English, Hebrew does not have a neuter pronoun. Coupled with the transmission of biblical texts through a patriarchal culture, masculine pronouns serve to refer to any human being in general (in the singular form) or a mixed group of males and females (in the plural form). Because our culture is more egalitarian, and *Living through Pain* makes no distinction between male and female readers, I have tried wherever possible to find genderless ways to render Hebrew pronouns, in keeping with the sense of the text. Failing in that, and trying both to avoid clumsy pairing of gender-specific pronouns and to communicate the profoundly personal tone of individual psalms, I have chosen to alternate the gender of the psalmists' voices in my discussion.

We confront a similar problem in references to God. Lacking a Hebrew neuter, and reflecting its patriarchal roots, biblical texts chose masculine forms where pronouns were necessary. However, biblical texts also passionately declare the impossibility of limiting God to a particular image; and with respect to gender, the whole corpus of biblical texts begins with reference to female, equally as male, likeness to God (Gen 1:27). Translators, then, face a thorny problem. Although I think the sense of biblical texts is served best by eschewing pronouns in reference to God in favor of simply "God," doing so mars the poetry of the psalms, to my ears. Consequently, with reservation and some concern, I have chosen to use the masculine pronoun in English where the same appears in the Hebrew in reference to God.

Issues of translation aside, I am interested in understanding something of the various shapes and textures of pain, what it is and what it does, and in promoting the productive and satisfying life of a whole person, even in the context of pain. The Bible is not the only voice on pain. Because pain as a whole-person event is a universal human experience, it is an object of interest and concern for every religious tradition. The first of Buddhism's "Four Noble Truths," and the one that drives the others, is that all life involves suffering. That the word *dukha*, here translated "suffering," means more than the pain of injury to include the sense of discontent and impermanence is instructive. To be whole/healed is to engage fully in one's present situation, to be alive as body, mind, and spirit in relation to others in the very real and ever-changing circumstances of one's life.

I begin with the problems of pain in an attempt to plumb the depths and wander the widths of this complicated human experience. In the first chapter, I briefly address aspects of pain-as-problem, including the toll it takes on individuals and society financially and otherwise, as well as the problems defining and describing pain. Considering pain-as-problem in these ways, I attempt not only to introduce the general necessity of taking the problem seriously and seriously seeking viable means of managing pain but also to underscore the particularity of pain—its radically personal nature and the manner in which psyche and spirit as well as body are involved in the experience. Finally, in the process of considering pain-as-problem, I attempt to introduce the idea that despite the individuality of pain, it also is influenced by and affects the sufferer's greater social context.

In chapter 2, I explore the matter of meaning-making and pain. There are two sides to this. As a whole-person experience, pain is subject to one's interpretation of it; and pain presses people to interpret it. How one thinks about one's pain affects the experience. Consider the difference between the pain of childbirth and the pain of torture. The pain is excruciating in both cases. However, in the first case, the pain is associated with the joyful event of bringing life, one's own child, into the world. It is anticipated and known to be of limited duration. In the second case, the pain is associated with terror and destruction, frequently compounded by knowing that one might also cause harm to one's family and/or community and by the ignorance of when and how long the torture will be. In addition to the matter of one's interpretation affecting one's experience of pain; pain also frequently demands an interpretation of its meaning and purpose. If one is religious, questions about divine power, justice, and love crowd to the front. In chapter 2, I concentrate especially on this aspect of meaning-making and pain, how pain drives people to ask questions about why they are suffering. I describe some of the ways in which people answer such questions and contemplate the implications of these answers both for the experience of pain in particular and for the more general matter of theology.

Chapter 3 introduces the Psalms with some information about their historical background and literary characteristics, and it briefly introduces the six psalms that I consider in detail in chapters 4–9. Because this book is not only for biblical scholars, I assume that many readers have little or no background in a study of the Bible. I also assume that many readers are not "religious," or if they are, are not necessarily Jewish or Christian. Consequently, in chapter 3, I attempt to explain both a little about the psalms, in general, and how it is that they have such power for Jews and Christians. In the process, I hope that readers will appreciate something about biblical texts as a part of our cultural heritage and also something about how they influence the people who consider them to be authoritative.

With chapter 4, I begin a close reading and discussion of six psalms, in particular. In these chapters, I do not try to show how these psalms might be applied for certain kinds of pain or certain circumstances of pain. Neither do I attempt to convince readers that they are answers to the kinds of existential or theological questions that pain may drive a person to ask. Instead, I invite readers to consider these psalms in light of different aspects of the experience of pain, and in so doing, engage with the psalmists in the process of wrestling with, asking about, and seeking to live through the experience of pain. In other words, each chapter is an invitation to move with the psalmist through his or her pain, experiencing the anguish, search for resolution, and personal transformations that each psalm represents.

The psalms that I consider, Psalms 6, 22, 38, 69, 88, and 102, share in common several things. They are voices out of pain, not thoughts on pain or hypothetical ideas about pain management; they represent a sense of self that is not neatly divided body from mind from spirit from community; and they are dynamic, reflecting not only pain's ever-changing nature but also the fact that we are always changing, too. In reading these psalms, I discuss different aspects of the experience of pain as the different psalms tell. These include the relationship between the pained person and his or her community, ways in which sufferers attempt to make sense of their pain, and the despair and darkness that great and sustained pain frequently elicits. They also include the power of changing how one thinks about one's pain and pain in the face of death.

In our reading, we witness the engagement of a whole person—body, mind, spirit, and community, in the dynamic of pain. In so doing, we engage in process—the process of candidly recognizing the reality of one's pain and responding with the authenticity of a unique, multi-faceted, whole person. The psalms move and we as readers move with them, contemplating the manner in which a person in pain grapples with questions of meaning, duration, and purpose. The psalmists do not all finally declare relief from their pain, or development from pain to a pain-free state. Instead, they demonstrate aspects of the experience and tell different ways of handling it. By paying attention, reading, and so getting involved with them, we have occasion to think about how to live fully through pain. The psalms do not tell us how to manage pain,

although sometimes they show us some of how a particular person (the psalmist) does so. The value of reading
them as we do here is in our engagement with them as fel-
low seekers who may yield insights into our own quest to
live as integrated selves, healthy even in the midst of pain.
We are less alone in our pain with such companions, and
the relief of loneliness may itself help mitigate the pain.

In my reading, I have frequently come across an ancient
story about a mother who cannot accept that her child is
dead. She brings him to the home of a holy man and asks
for medicine to cure him. Instead of trying to convince her
that the child is dead or otherwise instruct her in "getting
over it," the man tells her to get the necessary medicine by
obtaining a mustard seed from a home that has not known
suffering or death. As the woman goes from house to
house she discovers that everyone experiences pain, and
in the process, she finds the "medicine" that heals her
grief. There are at least a couple of different versions of
this story. In one version, she simply learns that death and
the pain of loss is universal. In another version, the
woman actually helps others, supporting them in their
grief and aiding them in the practical problems they face
after the loss of a family member. In both cases, her pain is
mitigated; and she participates in the community in a
manner that facilitates their healing, too. Reading the
psalms as we do in this book reveals that sometimes *we* are
"good medicine."[6]

I distinguish between curing and healing. I understand
curing to refer to a condition wherein persons no longer
have any of the signs or symptoms of whatever illness,
pain, or injury troubled them. To be cured, then, is in a
sense to return to a former state of being. Healing, on the
other hand, happens in any and all acts of making whole.
Healing involves the integration of all aspects of a per-

son—physical, psychological, spiritual, and social within that person's present context. It is no more the return to a previous state than it is the anticipation of a future one. It is rather to be a whole person fully engaged in the very real circumstances of one's present condition. People can be cured without being healed; and people can experience healing without being cured.[7] This book is not about curing pain. I cannot do that any more than the holy man could bring the woman's son back to life. However, this book is an invitation to engage a process. It is a tool for the reader to realize his or her own healing and to facilitate the healing of others.

1

Problems with Pain

~

"All life is suffering." —*Buddha*

It is not enough to say simply that pain is a problem, despite the frustrating combination of pain's prevalence and the scope of our ignorance about its causes and treatments. Pain elicits different kinds of problems. In this first chapter, I briefly describe three aspects of pain-as-problem: the problem *of* pain (its personal and social costs including difficulties with treatment), the problem *defining* pain (reflecting its variety and our developing understanding of its systemic/whole-person nature), and the problem *describing* pain (which contributes to difficulties managing it). Although there is considerable overlap between these categories, I treat each under a separate heading; as we learn more about each one, aspects of their interrelationships will become self-evident.

The first section, titled "The Price of Pain," lays the groundwork for appreciating the magnitude of pain's effects both personally and nationally and how these costs are related to difficulties with identification and treatment. My discussion of the issue is in no way comprehensive; rather, through pieces of pieces of the whole, I attempt to portray the greater general problem *of* pain. That is, I identify and briefly discuss a few characteristics and examples of the individual and social cost of pain in an effort to give a sense of the extent and kind of this aspect of pain's problematic nature. The second section, "The Myth of Two Pains,"[1] addresses that aspect of pain-as-problem concerned with *defining* pain. The tenacious, dominant model of understanding pain as a purely physical event is not without its critics. Noting how problematic that simplistic model has been, I discuss challenges to it and review some other ways that people try to categorize and define pain in an effort to account for pain's systemic/whole-person nature. Again, without a comprehensive analysis of all of the various responses to it, I suggest there is growing appreciation for the manner in which pain is perceived and affected by the great variety and complex relationships that compose an individual and dynamic self. Finally, the problem of *describing* pain merits its own space for investigation and discussion because of its relationships both to the problem of pain and to the problem *defining* pain. I introduce this topic in the section titled "Hard to Tell." Describing pain is a critical piece in the puzzle of addressing and alleviating pain; yet it is complicated not only by the difficulty others have understanding a sufferer's pain, but also by the sufferer's own understanding of his or her pain. In the process of considering these three general categories of the problems that attend pain, and the implications of them, the span of our inquiry broadens. Such expansion makes room for possibilities to take shape that allow for a better understanding of pain and ultimately for managing pain in ways that promote the rich development of individual lives.

The Price of Pain

I am not a mechanic, so when my car refuses to operate properly, I am at a loss. All plans leap out the window like

scared cats, and I am left holding the weight of my responsibilities, a burden that grows heavier with the knowledge
that it will probably cost me a great deal of time and
money to correct whatever is wrong with my car. Who
knows how much of each—time and money—and who
knows what's wrong anyway? My stomach sinks further.
I live within walking distance of the university where I
teach and of shops where I can buy necessities; but I have
not planned for this car trouble, and I find that its effects
are far-reaching. Then I am reminded of the student,
absent from class, who came to my office to explain that
her car had broken down while she was driving her four
year-old to daycare before heading to school. A bit
peeved, I knew that what she had missed was irreplaceable—a lecture organized by a topic and several themes
(not a document from which I read aloud), discussion,
and questions. The best she could do was talk to someone
in the class and get some notes about what we did there.
Now I remember how distressed she was and can imagine
how difficult it must be to deal with the work of parenting,
being a student, negotiating financial responsibilities, and
trying to fit in important social and recreational activities
when a basic resource is compromised. Although it would
not have changed the fact that we could not make up for
her loss, I am sorry that I dismissed the student so quickly,
sorry that I did not listen more closely.

Pain is a bit like that. We make plans, expecting things
to go along in a predictable manner, applying ourselves to
the tasks at hand, many of which are already stressful and
demanding. Then it comes—an ankle twisted, carpal tun-
nel syndrome, crippling lower back pain—and all bets are
off. Welcome to the problem *of* pain. Every year, millions
of people are unable to do their jobs on account of pain,
resulting in billions of dollars of lost work. In other words,

the problem of pain is reflected partly in significant financial and social costs, and recent studies suggest that
despite improvements in health care, such costs do not
appear to be decreasing.

According to the former surgeon general, David
Satcher, "the cost of pain reaches $100 billion annually
from, among other causes, lost workdays and unnecessary
hospitalizations."[2] A recent article published in the *Journal
of the American Medical Association* (*JAMA*) notes that
between August 1, 2001, and July 30, 2002, "thirteen percent of the total workforce experienced a loss in productive time during a 2-week period due to a common pain
condition."[3] Although the financial rewards of disability
motivate some people to claim debilitating pain when they
do not have such pain, the *JAMA* study notes "the majority
(76.6%) of the lost productive time was explained by
reduced performance while at work and not work
absence."[4] The American Chronic Pain Association
(ACPA), a non-profit organization with 400 chapters
worldwide that provides support to people in pain, notes
that 86 million Americans are unable to work because of
their pain. Comparison with earlier studies does not indicate improvement over the past decade. Culling information from studies done in 1990 and 1991, Maryann Bates,
an anthropologist interested in the varying ways that different cultures experience, express, and manage pain,
notes that the then-estimated cost each year of chronic
pain in the United States, factoring in medications, disability compensation, and lost wages, was between fifty
and ninety billion dollars.[5] "Pain accounts for over 70 million office visits each year to physicians in the United
States" is Dennis C. Turk's sobering introduction to his
published 1993 article.[6]

An article published in June 2003 reports the results of a study of the costs that fibromyalgia, just one among many kinds of chronic pain, incurs for employers. By way of example, I cite that study here. Although little is known about specific causes and less about treatment, fibromyalgia (a name that refers to pain in the body's fibers) originates in connective tissues such as tendons, ligaments, and muscles, and causes varying degrees and kinds of pain, along with considerable fatigue. David X. Cifu, whose research and skills as a physical medicine and rehabilitation physician have earned him an international reputation, notes that finally fibromyalgia is "just a word" that has come to apply to a wide range of mysterious and debilitating pains that hijack the lives of its sufferers.[7] We know little more than that the pain is real.

Six researchers for Eli Lilly and Company undertook an inquiry of fibromyalgia's costs having noted, "Fibromyalgia (FM) is characterized by widespread pain that can lead to significant patient disability, complex management decisions for physicians, and economic burden on society." They used data from a Fortune 100 manufacturer reflecting claims associated with fibromyalgia that carried both "direct (i.e., medical and pharmaceutical claims) and indirect (i.e., disability claims and imputed absenteeism) costs." Their findings show that people claiming to suffer from fibromyalgia cost about two and a half times more each year than other employees ($5,945 vs. $2,486). Furthermore, "the prevalence of disability was twice as high among FM employees than overall employees." Perhaps most sobering, "for every dollar spent on FM specific claims, the employer spent another $57 to $143 on additional direct and indirect costs." They concluded, "Hidden costs of disability and comorbidities greatly increase the true burden of FM. Regardless of the clinical understanding of FM, when a claim for FM is present, considerable costs are involved."[8] Publication of these findings in the international, peer reviewed *Journal of Rheumatology* suggests that the research is credible and the findings accurate.

With hyperbole and fact, pain has been described as a very expensive matter. The ACPA calls pain "the number one cause of adult disability in the United States." It has been labeled an "epidemic." Steven F. Brena identified it as such as early as 1978 with the book titled *Chronic Pain: America's Hidden Epidemic.*[9] More recently Kathryn Weiner, serving as the executive director of the American Academy of Pain Management, did so with her article, "Pain is an Epidemic."[10] In September 2003, *US Newswire* quoted former Health and Human Services Secretary Dr. Louis Sullivan as saying, "Untreated pain, tragically, is an epidemic in the United States." A survey conducted for Ortho-McNeil Pharmaceutical in 1999 and published under the title *National Pain Survey* estimated that about 24 percent of people from the United States (approximately 48 million) suffer from some type of chronic pain. Results of the survey tell that 42 percent of pain sufferers are so disabled by the pain that they are unable to work, and 63 percent are unable to perform satisfactorily the tasks of day-to-day living.[11]

There are problems with each of these claims. One could argue that the ACPA's claim concerning adult disability is misleading because other claims of disability are of a different category, or, more precisely, a subcategory. That is, an injury causing disability often continues to be painful, so how is the cause of disability identified, by injury or by pain? Similarly, one could argue that the term *epidemic* is vague, not defined as exceeding a specific number of cases. Furthermore, one could say that the survey's results should be considered with suspicion, because a pharmaceutical company, which stands to gain money from the development and prescription of pain medications, conducted it. Indeed, it is possible to undermine each of these claims; yet finally, despite problems of terminology and interest, evidence from the myriad, thriving places and people defined by the promise of alleviating pain, not to say from our own individual experiences, certainly suggests that pain is a widespread, and even growing problem. This is especially provocative in the face of remarkable improvements in health care.

There seems, especially in the case of problematic chronic pain, to be a counterintuitive correlation between treatment options and cost. While some of the new techniques of treatment are astonishingly successful in alleviating pain, many are not, or are so only for a brief period of time; and sometimes the subsequent pain is worse than the pain that impelled the sufferer to seek relief in the first place. Consequently, for people with considerable resources and suffering intractable pain, the price of attempting to alleviate their pain becomes exorbitant as they shuttle from place to place trying treatment after treatment. As the record of their treatments grow, these people come to be called "thick folder patients." One such patient, although publicly portrayed as robustly healthy, was John F. Kennedy. In 2002, presidential historian Robert Dallek was granted access to Kennedy's medical files. Based on his research, Dallek tells the story of an ambitious man who, with "iron-willed fortitude," kept hidden from the public a lifetime of illness and extraordinary pain.[12] Ronald Melzack and Patrick Wall, pioneers in the field of pain management and highly respected among the greater medical community for moving pain out of its secondary or tertiary place behind injury and into a field of its own, wrote, "Kings and presidents are in considerable danger of rigorous curative therapies terminated only by the closure of the coffin lid."[13] Kennedy's experience demonstrates the truth behind their observation. Indeed, with virtually limitless resources, the continuing search for pain relief can be endless and consequently, tremendously taxing.

I do not mean to suggest that we should eschew attempts to alleviate pain; on the contrary, it is incumbent upon us to provide pain relief with proven results and to continue to explore new ways to treat pain. Reviewing the wide range of medical treatment options and issues of access is not within the scope of this book.[14] However, by recognizing that pain continues to be and is increasingly a problem of its own, we admit that techniques for dealing with it must involve a variety of approaches, some of which simply equip the sufferer to apply skills that enable him or her to live productively with the pain. The rise in "multidisciplinary" pain clinics demonstrates the existence of such an attitude among the medical community, as they seek to apply the knowledge and techniques of a variety of disciplines to the problem of a patient's pain. Because so many clinics have developed so recently and they are defined by the diversity of staff and treatments, to date there is not a consistent standard to the methods and administration of these clinics. They vary widely in approach and success.

The number and diversity of these clinics attests to the scope of the problem of pain. Pain management as a goal unto itself, not simply in association with other diagnoses, is a very recent development. Despite the early importance of Melzack and Wall's work, Melzack credits John Bonica with creating the whole field of pain inquiry and

analysis; and Bonica did so by appreciating the importance of drawing on a wide variety of approaches to the
treatment of pain. The rise in groups defined by their concern with managing and alleviating pain matches the
growth in multidisciplinary pain clinics. The International
Association for the Study of Pain (IASP) was begun by
John Bonica in 1972 and as of August 2003 it boasts 6,744
members from 107 countries. The American Academy of
Pain Management, with membership estimated at 6,000,
competes with the IASP for designation as the largest
pain organization in the United States; the numbers indicate a tie.[15] Both define themselves by the variety of people involved in the search to alleviate pain on pain's own
terms. The breakdown of membership by discipline in the
Academy of Pain Management shows that physicians
compose the largest group (61 percent, of which the
largest subgroup are anesthesiologists [37 percent]), followed by chiropractors, mental health professionals, den-
tists and "others" in equal numbers, podiatrists, nurses,
and lastly equal numbers of pharmacists and physical
therapists.

The existence and growth of groups, such as the ACPA
mentioned above, further supports the fact that pain continues to be a very real problem for many individuals
despite both increasing treatment options and the development of a multidisciplinary approach within the general
area of medicine. The Association among other groups
concerned with the problem of pain is unusual in its composition and mission. While most organizations reflect the
valuable work of medical professionals, academic and
clinical, the ACPA is defined by its "lay" involvement.
That is, its core membership is people suffering from pain,
and its primary form of organization is small support
groups, wherein members can share confidentially the

many facets of their experiences dealing with pain. In the process, they not only have a forum in which to tell their own stories candidly, but they also can support and encourage others in pain. Begun in 1980, the Association has grown to include more than 400 chapters in countries spanning four continents. It has developed an educational outreach campaign called Partners for Understanding Pain, which includes over sixty groups and/or institutions committed to pain management.

Another aspect of the problem of pain's high cost that I will mention only briefly is the legal one. Because pain is so little understood, physicians who attempt to alleviate their patients' excruciating pain with powerful narcotics sometimes face suspicion, even arrest, by law enforcement officials concerned about the abuse of such medications. The attempt to correct misunderstandings about abuse of and addiction to narcotics by people in pain and the medical doctors who treat them makes the National Foundation for the Treatment of Pain (NFTP) unique among peer groups. Recognizing that undertreatment of pain is a very real problem, not simply because individuals suffer unnecessarily but also because of the financial and social costs in lost work, the NFTP is, among other things, committed to defending physicians wrongfully prosecuted for prescribing narcotics appropriate to the chronic pain that their patients present.[16]

While statistics and knowledge of the development and growth of organizations such as the IASP and ACPA can be helpful in illustrating the nature and scope of the problem of pain, we all know that they don't tell the whole story—the story of individual lives disrupted and torn in many ways and on different levels. Therein lies another aspect of the costly problem of pain. It is not possible to distinguish the effects of pain on an individual's life from other events/aspects of that same life. Pain prohibits a father from lifting his child, prevents a woman from hiking with friends. Pain makes it impossible to change a light bulb, ride the subway to work, walk the dog, and do the laundry. Pain demands the brain's attention, arresting the concentration necessary to get the work of a desk job done and inhibiting the caution necessary to protect from further injury in construction work. It makes a high school student seem ill-prepared for and uninterested in class and makes a parent impatient and self-absorbed when her three-year-old misbehaves or heads for trouble. Pain can make it impossible to listen to a friend's story of loss, or comfort an elderly uncle worried about the effects of his aging. The examples are as endless and the effects in each life are as intertwined as Penelope's tapestry. The compromises to any individual life that pain demands and its disruptive effects on other relationships create conditions of self-doubt and depression, low self-esteem and a sense of purposelessness. They contribute to a vicious cycle of feeling bad, feeling bad about feeling bad, and feeling worse. Furthermore, the "feeling" is done on all levels—mental, physical, social, and spiritual—all of which contribute to the perception of pain. I discuss briefly below three kinds of pain (lower back pain, neuropathy, and complex regional pain) in an effort to illustrate both the life-disrupting nature of pain and the range of ways it is identified and felt.

Lower back pain is one of the most common pain problems today. Headaches are the other most common; but while headaches come and go, lower back pain tends to be constant. Although its reality is undeniable to the person suffering, finding the/a specific source of lower back pain is notoriously difficult to do. The following medical explanation, provided by the Resource Center of the first

Department of Pain and Palliative Care in the United States, at Beth Israel Hospital in New York City, is telling. The explanation begins by describing possible causes for back pain in unsurprising, pedestrian ways: injury to the nerves, arthritis, and problems with the disks in and of the vertebrae. Then it grows more complicated, noting that usually there is some combination of these things, and further that "stress and other psychological factors play a part in how severe the pain is, how long it lasts, and how much it interferes with your life."[17] The authors add that those suffering lower back pain often cannot move in the most basic ways that non-sufferers take for granted. For example, lower back pain often prohibits people from bending, leaning, or standing up straight. Sufferers sometimes describe pain running down the leg, even into the foot; and others say that they feel tingling or numbness, like a limb that is falling asleep. The experts add simply, "many patients can't function normally because of the pain" and note finally a high incidence of depression, insomnia, and general weariness.

Neuropathic pain is the type of chronic pain that is the most difficult to treat, according to medical researcher, Catherine Bushnell, at McGill University. Causing pain that is sometimes local, sometimes general, this nerve problem seems to have no single identifiable cause, and its felt effects are as wide-ranging. The brush of clothes or wind can trigger terrible episodes. Even its name belies its mystery. All that can be said about it is that something is wrong with the nerves, hence "neuro-pathic," by which the brain is overrun by pain messengers eager to communicate a crisis that sometimes is not there. Although the nerves may repair and regenerate themselves, the pain requires attention on its own terms. Observing that untreated pain simply gets worse in intensity and duration, Bushnell is not alone in advocating early treatment of the pain with medication dosages equal to the level of pain. But she is especially motivated by the link between psychological processes and the experience of pain. Indeed, both those suffering pain and their caretakers have noted that a person's thinking and the degree of pain she or he suffers are directly related. Distractions alleviate pain. Because her research demonstrates such a link, Dr. Bushnell asserts that the connection between body and mind must be taken more seriously.[18]

While lower back pain is most often related to tissue injury (if a cause can be determined), and neuropathy is due to nerve injury, "complex regional pain syndrome" seems to embody pain's rejection of even these most general identifications. For one thing, complex regional pain syndrome (CRPS) is sometimes called by one of two other names: "causalgia," which reflects the fact that CRPS could follow on injury to nerves; or "reflex sympathetic dystrophy," which reflects the fact that CRPS could follow on non-nerve related injury. Although physicians agree that the syndrome follows some kind of injury, the injury need not be serious and sometimes patients don't remember any previous injury at all. It can hurt anywhere, though it is most common in arms and legs; and it can express itself in all sorts of ways, including sweating and swelling. Sometimes it travels and sometimes it stays in a particular area of the body; sometimes the pain gets worse and sometimes it goes away. There is no single method for curing it. That CRPS can cause depression, shaking, insomnia, and wasting away of skin and bones, among many other things, makes it easy to imagine how disrupting this condition can be to anyone who suffers from it.

The wide range of ways in which pain can be felt and expressed is reflected in the wide range of effects it can have on a person's life. Nessa Coyle, a registered nurse who has logged many hours of bedside work, culled from patients' medical charts their own words for their experience of pain and its effects. In organizing their quotations, she determined the following categories to be appropriate: despair, loneliness, vulnerability; disappointments; bewilderment; loss; worry (about being a burden and about finances); fear (of disability, abandonment, death, night); and general weariness. Coyle reports what we have come to suspect that pain is immediate and overwhelming and can result in a loss of hope and an exhausted spirit.[19]

Introducing only these three—lower back pain, neuropathy, and complex regional pain syndrome—which represent both kind and category of pain out of the plethora that people may suffer, suggests how problematic addressing the pain can be. Sometimes people prefer not to treat it at all. Indeed, because pain can warn us against activity that might cause further damage, some sufferers assume their pain to be the sign of some other problem that needs to be addressed—that it is telling something important and so should not be silenced. While this is true of some kinds of pain, no pain is "good" if it continues too long. Furthermore, pain is seldom as helpful a source of information guarding against further injury as we might hope. There is not a consistent, one-to-one correspondence of pain and bodily damage. Think of the soldier who felt no pain when injured in the heat of battle, or by contrast, the absence of apparent injury in most people with lower back pain.[20] Consider also the lack of pain as a fatal cancer develops (which later during treatment and in its final stages can bring excruciating pain).

Related to the problem of assuming that pain is directly associated with injury and so should be endured as long as it takes to identify and cure the primary injury, is the problem of telling pain to others. Many in pain do not want to burden others with unpleasant complaints, anger, and despair. Indeed, healthy people often would rather not hear about another's pain, for several reasons. For one thing, it is not fun. This can be an understatement with terrible implications, as Sophocles's *Philoctetus* dramatizes. In this play, dating to the late fifth century BCE, the protagonist suffers a snake bite on his foot that grows infected and is excruciating in its pain. Unable to do anything except complain, he is abandoned by his shipmates on a rocky island. Not only is it unpleasant to hear complaints simply because they are complaints, but also in the case of pain, the listener often feels powerless to help. And of course the person in pain knows that he or she is not good company, yet has difficulty not thinking about (and so talking about) his or her pain. Elaine Scarry, whose ground-breaking book *The Body in Pain* investigates how pain can be a force of either destruction or creation, notes, "Before destroying language, [pain] first monopolizes language, becomes its only subject: complaint [. . .] becomes the exclusive mode of speech."[21] A person in great pain frequently tells of complete preoccupation with it, a constant monitoring of this or that activity, posture, or attitude and how it affects the experience of pain. Although distraction sometimes alleviates pain, finding distraction that "works" is difficult and nearly always temporary. Hope renewed and dashed in cycles contributes to the frustration, which contributes to the preoccupation with pain, which hijacks speech until it is nothing more than complaint. It is a downward spiraling process that makes relief from the telling more difficult, with grave personal and social results.

While the listener may feel powerless to relieve the suffering of her friend, simply listening can do much to help;

and maybe that is partly why the person in pain feels so compelled to tell of it. But pain is infectious. It has a catchy character, making it difficult to get a hearing among the healthy. Not only can its report make the listener feel a bit down herself, but sometimes otherwise healthy people report the onset of symptoms similar to the person in pain. Marni Jackson writes of her experience researching shingles, which led to what seemed for all intents and purposes to be an early stage of its development in her.[22] Not that this always happens, but one wonders if the basic aversion to hearing about pain when one is free of it, is partly due to a subconscious concern about a risk of contracting it. Finally, it may be that hearing about pain reminds us that it is not an escapable experience. Living without pain is a temporary state.

In short, pain is the cause of great financial cost both to individuals and to the greater society dependent on such individuals' contributions. The price of pain is incalculable when one considers also the personal and social toll that pain exacts as it disintegrates the sufferer herself/himself and fractures relationships of all kinds.

The Myth of Two Pains[23]

This brief review of the problem *of* pain, due to its wide-reaching effects and the interdisciplinary, systemic nature of pain, suggests that it eludes easy definition. For one thing, there is wide variety in pain's expression, not only in terms of the places where it might be felt (localized in a limb, or primary to an internal site, for example) but also in pain's quality (piercing, dull, burning, etc.) and intensity (annoying to excruciating). Pain is thus dynamic. Complicating the matter yet more, we have noted that pain cannot be isolated from the whole of a person. Pain is systemic, affecting and affected by all aspects of the individual suffering, including his or her social and cultural context.

This great variety would seem to suggest that one cannot precisely define pain. Yet, without launching immediately into the bleak impossibility of ever doing so, there are some things we can indeed say about it. No matter how much we theorize and attempt to trace the transfer of information along nerve pathways to the meaning-making matter of gray cells in the brain, setting one's hand on an open flame hurts. Those who study pain in the clinic and lab have identified a complex system of nerve interaction that communicates such pain to the brain and so can reduce the extent of the injury caused by something like fire. Descartes was onto this with his proposal in 1664 of understanding pain like a bell-ringing process signaling injury, which he illustrated with the drawing of a single path from (injured) limb to brain. This simple explanation works pretty well for defining acute pain. However, as briefly demonstrated and discussed above, there are many exceptions to the explanation and many more cases for which such an explanation is not at all accurate.

Daniel Carr, a physician, the editor-in-chief of *Pain: Clinical Updates* (a publication of the IASP), and executive director of TOP MED (Topics in Pain Medicine, an initiative to educate medical students about pain), reflects on today's more sophisticated understanding of the complex system of the body's communicating pain and hints at its more-than-the-body nature. He notes, "Pain is a dynamic process that involves actions at multiple sites ranging from the peripheral nociceptor to the genome of cells within the central nervous system to the patient's psychosocial milieu."[24] Less a definition than a description, Carr's explanation accounts for both the immediate pain that injury may cause and the affect that society and culture can have on a person's experience of pain. That he includes "ranging" in this description allows for the every-thing-in-between, the complicated nature of a whole person, composed of myriad and dynamic interrelated aspects, which makes defining pain so difficult. Jennifer Pearson, who incorporates her clinical experience into medical school courses at the University of Minnesota, notes that to practice medicine as a "healer's art" is to rec-ognize with one's patients the warp and woof of life. She observes that because traditional, modern medicine downplays the effects of a person's emotional and spiritual experiences on physiological processes, it is ill equipped to handle the problem of chronic pain.[25]

Until very recently, our so-called Western society (and its attendant medical system) has considered pain as a purely physical phenomenon. Certainly, the connection of physiological tissue damage to the experience of pain is undeniable; but even in a seemingly straightforward injury, the complicated interconnection of the self's many facets is evident. In the case of a car accident, for example, many people report feeling no pain until some time after the event, though suffering severe injuries such as lacera-tions, broken bones, and even burns. Another example is the average Joes or Janes who rise to heroic heights in helping others incur injury that they report had no atten-dant pain until the danger was past. And again, think of the high incidence of "phantom limb" pain among amputees (even among people born without limbs), a fre-quently excruciating experience notoriously difficult to relieve because the site that the brain thinks is injured is not there. By contrast, there are those who claim relief from pain by apparently inviting it. "Cutters," for exam-ple, engage in self-injurious behavior, drawing their own blood, in order paradoxically to feel better. Especially common among women, cutting is a means of relieving what feels like a deeper and greater pain than any that the lacerations elicit. Marni Jackson proposes, "someone who inscribes her body like this is also writing. She's just chosen the harshest medium possible for telling her story."[26] Taking the phenomenon yet further to actual pleasure, think of the popularity of sadomasochism among sexual adventurers for whom pain is a crucial part of the erotic experience. These and many other, less dramatic examples, such as the power of entertaining distraction to relieve pain, demonstrate the impossibility of separating the body from the mind when it comes to pain. Yet, perhaps because it is much more difficult to understand and implies that pain often resists simple pharmacological or surgical treatment, considering pain within the context of a person's whole self is less common than treating it as an isolated physical event.

Indeed, the attempt to distinguish what we call *body* and *mind* continues to persist and to inform the ways in which we understand and talk about pain. David B. Morris, in his study of the relationship of culture to one's experience of pain, calls this "the myth of two pains." He notes the tenacity of this idea that pain is either physical or mental, and observes, "Between these two different events we seem to imagine a gulf so wide and deep that it might as well be filled by a sea that is impossible to navigate."[27] Morris's effort to demonstrate the role of culture in one's experience of pain and so allow a variety of voices, past and present, to lend insight and even meaning to one's experience of pain is an attempt to bridge that gulf. I agree with him that misunderstandings about pain as a purely biochemical experience are not limited to the field of medicine, but permeate our society's thinking, largely informed by a scientific worldview.

As a matter of fact, these misunderstandings seem to persist more strongly and are more fixed outside of the field of medicine than within it. Already in 1965, Melzack and Wall put forward a revolutionary new model in the understanding of pain perception. Their "gate-control" theory suggests that both physical and mental processes are in operation, indeed interact with one another, to inform a person's perception of pain.[28] Specifically, they observed that while there does indeed seem to be a process of communication from the site of injury to the brain, there is a simultaneous direction of communication *away from* the brain that affects and modifies the former information. Subsequent to Melzack and Wall's work, people increasingly recognized that despite pain's immediate sense as a bodily phenomenon, its intensity, duration, and interpretation depend on a whole-person process. Indeed, Ephrem Fernandez recently published a book-length report of studies in clinical psychology describing an inextricable link between emotions and pain.[29] Naomi Eisenberger has shown a demonstrable connection between social rejection/loss and pain by noting their effect on the same brain center. The study made national news by linking a sense of heartache with physiological measurement of its effect.[30]

John E. Sarno has made headlines and continues to be an outspoken and controversial figure in the medical field of pain management for his theory that nearly all back pain is the body's way of hiding painful emotions, particularly anger. The result, he suggests, is a kind of tension that produces a physiological reaction that "leads to painful muscle spasm and nerve pain."[31] Treatment, then, is a matter of the patient thinking of his or her pain in emotional terms. Douglas Hoffman, an orthopedic physician, found Sarno's theory credible after both personal experience of relief from problematic pain and extensive research involving the history, demographics, and efficacy of back pain treatment. Hoffman now offers interested patients guided treatment, and he reports remarkable success, further demonstrating the problems of defining pain in purely physiological terms.[32]

In an effort to define pain, in general, the Resource Center at Beth Israel's Department of Pain and Palliative Care, discussed earlier, proposes that it be defined as "an unpleasant feeling that may or may not be related to an injury, illness, or other bodily trauma," but adds that finally "pain is complex and differs from person to person."[33] In an attempt to standardize terminology associated with pain, the IASP proposes defining pain as "an unpleasant sensory and emotional experience associated with actual or potential tissue damage, or described in terms of such damage." While they are careful to define it in a manner that privileges its physical nature, they admit that it is not simply a biophysical matter. "It is unquestionably a sensation in a part or parts of the body, but it is also always unpleasant and therefore also an emotional experience."[34] Although this admission does not seem to allow for the possibility that what they term *emotions* may actually inform the pain experience in all manners of its expression, the IASP's definition of pain includes a note that it is "always subjective." Together with comments including the vague "in terms of such damage," pain's emotional aspect, and its subjective character, the IASP has opened the door to a definition of pain that makes the physical aspect, which reigns in their present definition, only one among others.

In general, pain is defined first by reference to one of two categories—acute and chronic. Identifying acute pain is usually easy, associated with a particularly memorable injury, and is often just as easy to treat. Partners for Understanding Pain (launched by the ACPA) explain, "Acute pain has a distinct beginning and end. The cause of acute pain is known and, as you heal, the pain will lessen and finally go away."[35] Chronic pain, by contrast, poses the greatest challenges and is the source of most of the problems identified and described in this book. Unfortunately, acute pain can become chronic pain simply by sticking around or recurring over time. Chronic pain is inconsistent. It varies from person to person, and its experience changes for the individual in pain, varying in intensity, kind, and even location.

The IASP has a whole "task force" devoted to the grinding duty of classifying kinds of chronic pain. A sample list of terms that appear frequently to describe types of chronic pain is itself dizzying: allodynia, analgesia, anesthesia dolorosa, causalgia, central pain, dysesthesia, hyperesthesia, hypoalgesia, hypoesthesia, neuralgia, neuritis, neuropathic pain, neuropathy, noxious stimulus, paresthesia, peripheral neurogenic pain, and peripheral neuropathic pain.[36] The list is an update from 1986, revealing the ever-changing nature of how we understand pain. Incidentally, the pain that Bushnell describes as the most difficult, neuropathic pain, is a newcomer to the list.

That the authors of the IASP's basic information about pain for lay readers finally admit that a patient's claim of pain should be accepted calls into question the attempt to distinguish physical from psychological pain.[37] Despite its complicating implications for understanding and treating pain, more and more people seem willing to acknowledge that the body and mind cannot be so clearly distinguished when it comes to pain. An article published in the IASP newsletter by Anthony K. P. Jones of the Manchester University's Rheumatic Diseases Centre, states, "The experience of pain can be defined only in terms of human consciousness. [. . .] Pain should not be equated with nociception."[38] Nevertheless, quantifying, much less documenting, the relationship is a notoriously difficult undertaking. In his book, Fernandez draws from over 750 references to identify and describe the connection between pain perception and "affects," such as anxiety, depression, and anger. In the course of his discussion, Fernandez notes the strengths and weaknesses of a variety of assessment instruments and suggests possibilities for future research.[39] One such area concerns the demographics of pain. Karen Berkley, a neurologist inquiring about differences between the ways in which women and men experience pain, writes of "biology's mutually modulatory factors," a tongue-twister that she explains includes "social, psychological, physiological, cellular, molecular, and genetic factors." All of these, she argues, are operative in an individual's experience of pain.[40] Such admission is shaping contemporary approaches to pain management, even though it complicates attempts to define pain.

Perhaps the unwillingness of Melzack and Wall to define pain definitively in 1973 and again in 1982 should still be the model. They do not argue that no definition is possible, but simply that a satisfactory one had not at that time been offered. They suggest, "pain may be defined in terms of a multidimensional space comprising several sensory and affective dimensions. The space comprises those subjective experiences which have both somatosensory and negative-affective components and that elicit behavior aimed at stopping the conditions that produce them."[41] Unusual at the time, people now are beginning to appreciate that pain is not a simple biophysical matter, but is inseparable from all facets of each individual, complex person with a particular history and within a particular cultural context. We are learning that pain cannot be isolated from psyche, spirit, and society. Pain is a whole-self event.

Consequently, it becomes difficult to distinguish pain from suffering. We usually attribute pain to bodily distress and suffering to the more generalized, multifaceted distress that I note here. Indeed, the two are related and therein lies our answer: they cannot finally be neatly separated. Although pain may start as what seems to be a simple biophysical experience, attending to its own developmental life, we soon see how it cannot be separated from psychological, spiritual, and social distress. Morris appeals to the genre of tragedy for instruction, explaining, "Suffering is a kind of damage that extends beyond the body to afflict the mind or soul or spirit too. [. . .] Tragedy expresses a twofold or circular wisdom: to understand pain you must understand suffering, and to understand suffering you must understand pain."[42]

That is, despite its physical manifestation, pain depends in part on the manner in which the pained person thinks about it. Indeed, another paradoxical aspect of pain is seemingly manic leaps between despair and elation, depression and confidence that people in pain experience. Because today's experience of pain is largely absent of the kind of meanings that it may have had or promoted in other cultural contexts,[43] the upside of these pairings is seldom as easily experienced as the downsides. Most people, especially those in chronic pain, suffer terrible depression as they struggle to find a source and consequent treatment for their pain; and many physicians report that a regular part of their treatment of chronic pain now includes antidepressants.[44] People in chronic pain frequently experience low self-esteem as the work and recreation they were accustomed to doing becomes difficult or impossible, and they may become angry at and resentful toward others who are pain-free. Sufferers frequently see their lives in uncontrollable disarray, often battling ailing relationships and a sense of worthlessness, even of being a burden on others.

These experiences are partly due to the narrow definition of pain as a theoretically curable physiological event, which leads many sufferers to circumscribe pain as an aberration in one's life. Arthur Frank, who promotes telling of one's pain as a therapeutic method (for the pained individual) and moral imperative (to help others in pain), writes of the tendency to employ a "restitution narrative."[45] This kind of self-story is based on an understanding of one's pain as a passing thing, due to illness or injury that will be cured and after which life will resume just like it did before the pain. Frank observes that this can be a helpful way to understand and deal with the problem of a definable, acute pain; but it can become a burden itself when the cure is elusive and the pain sustained. Other ways of thinking about pain in one's life become necessary in order that the suffering person live as well as possible, starting *now* and not at some point when the pain is past. I find much in Frank's work that is valuable for reintegrating the self that is struggling to deal with intractable pain. His general thesis that "bodies need voices" presumes that the experience of pain or illness is not only a part of that life but also that its effects can be managed and controlled.

Indeed, the manner in which one defines pain is part of one's experience of it; and the manner in which one describes pain in the context of one's whole life can actually shape the experience, indeed that life. That a definition of pain may finally be impossible to determine, once and for all, simply points to its subjectivity and systemic nature. It is not only a purely personal experience with as

many variations as there are people, but also inextricably
bound up in the complicated, multifaceted nature of each
individual life. Pain is dynamic, ever-changing with the
ever-changing nature of a person's life.

Hard to Tell

The difficulty of defining pain is reflected in the difficulty
of describing it. In her essay "On Being Ill," Virginia
Woolf wrote, "English, which can express the thoughts of
Hamlet and the tragedy of Lear, has no words for the
shiver and the headache. [. . .] The merest schoolgirl,
when she falls in love, has Shakespeare and Keats to
speak for her; but let a sufferer try to describe a pain in his
head to a doctor and language at once runs dry." Indeed,
the problem of describing pain may well be a part of its
definition, intrinsic to the nature of pain itself. The experience of pain is fundamentally subjective, depending as it
does on the many different aspects of a person's life, both
individual and social. There is, then, a consequent difficulty communicating one's pain to others. Pain, in its fracturing of an individual self—that is, of relationships
between the self's different aspects—also fractures that
person's relationship to others just as the impossibility of
clearly communicating the experience creates a gulf
between the sufferer and others. Indeed, while aspects of
an individual person have their own distinct characteristics and a person is undeniably distinct from others, pain
not only clarifies those distinctions but also widens the
gaps both between aspects of the self and between the self
and others. Difficulty describing pain adds insult to the
injury, yet it seems unavoidable. It is part of the nature of
pain itself. Elaine Scarry writes, "[pain's] resistance to
language is not simply one of its incidental or accidental
attributes but is essential to what it is."[46] The problem of

describing how such pain affects the sufferer is the focus of this section; and there are several facets to the problem.

For one thing, pain cruelly interferes with the ability to speak at all, at its most intense and terrifying levels reducing the sufferer to shrieks and groans. Related, the attempt to find the words to communicate a pain demonstrates its "as-if" nature. We describe pain in similes and metaphors, searching for likenesses among common experiences, images or senses that share in some way with this feeling that finally defies words. The McGill-Melzack Pain Questionnaire was developed to address just such a difficulty for medical practitioners attempting to understand the nature of their patients' complaints. One part has many adjectives, arranged in twenty categories, from which patients choose to describe the pain that they feel. Together with its two other parts, a descriptive scale from one to five of pain intensity and a drawing of the body on which the patient points to areas where he or she experiences pain, the McGill-Melzack Pain Questionnaire is the most widely used tool of its kind. Yet despite its length and detail, the questionnaire can only get a little closer to describing the fundamentally individual experience of pain. Pain is not distinct from the one who perceives it, and it is affected by that perception.

Another method that attempts to bridge the gap between the person in pain and those trying to help requires patients to rank their pain on a scale from zero to ten, zero being no pain and ten representing the worst pain imaginable. The technique of rating the intensity of pain according to a numerical scale is problematic for several reasons—desires to exaggerate or alternatively downplay pain; the subjectivity of the person asking; and the lack of decent comparisons. Think of how many times people describe pain as worse than they thought possible.

One wonders where on the scale terrific pain experienced before would rank. Sometimes new pain makes the previous seem less than one might have judged at the time. Furthermore, Melzack and Wall note that this method, and others like it, measure only intensity and liken the exercise to "specifying the visual world only in terms of light flux without regard to pattern, colour (sic), texture, and the many other dimensions of visual experience."[47] That there are variations on these questionnaires and other ones attests to the difficulty of describing pain. They also demonstrate the importance of trying. In other words, the attempt to describe pain is bound up with the continuing search to alleviate it.

It is, then, imperative not only that the person in pain attempt to communicate her experience but also that others work to understand it. There is something in this process that is basic to the quest to reintegrate a fractured self, and with that, to reintegrate that self into the greater community. In other words, other people are critical to the process, even, perhaps especially, at the level simply of witnesses present to the sufferer's process of definition and understanding despite an inherent inability fully to grasp the experience of another's pain. Scarry's description of the difficulty we have understanding another's pain, as something like trying to know a subterranean occurrence or invisible galaxy, is evocative and underscores the great gap between the one telling and the one hearing about pain. She concludes, "vaguely alarming yet unreal, laden with consequence yet evaporating before the mind because not available to sensory confirmation, [. . .] the pains occurring in other people's bodies flicker before the mind, then disappear."[48] Yet while the gulf of misunderstanding between the person in pain and others is wide, it need not be so fixed as Scarry implies. Managing pain and so reintegrating a fractured self depends partly on both the telling of pain and the recognition that those hearing cannot completely understand. The attentive witness of others can do much to help alleviate a person's pain as the sufferer seeks new understanding of herself as a whole life in relation to others; and such witness does not depend on perfectly comprehending the full nature of another's pain. But I am getting ahead of myself.

For the time being, it is enough to note a fundamental paradox: that pain is both simultaneously undeniable to the person experiencing it and unconfirmable for those hearing about it. In the medical field, this problem is sometimes expressed in a patient's reticence to report the pain at all. This poses definite problems of treatment frequently resulting in under-treatment of the pained patient. Recognizing such danger, the IASP cautions, "the inability to communicate verbally does not negate the possibility that an individual is experiencing pain and is in need of appropriate pain-relieving treatment."[49] Sometimes the patient may try to communicate the nature of his or her pain but does so incompletely and/or by means of what may seem to the medical practitioner to be gross tangents. All of us communicate using vocabulary and style tailored to our audience; the manner of describing pain is partly dependent on the society of which the sufferer is a part and by the cultural field(s) of both speaker and hearer. This can exacerbate the problem a patient faces communicating his or her pain if she or he is trying to use an unfamiliar language, for example, that of medicine. It is important that the physician encourage the person in pain to describe the experience in the manner most comfortable to the patient.

Furthermore, it is important that the medical practitioner also listen carefully to the patient's seeming tangents. The point of Turk's article, "Assess the Person, Not Just the Pain" is to underscore the fundamental subjectivity of pain, noting "It is highly unlikely that we will ever be able to evaluate pain without reliance on the individual's perceptions."[50] And recent studies demonstrate that different people feel what would seem to be the same pain differently. Robert Coghill of Wake Forest University in Winston-Salem, North Carolina, conducted brain scans on people whom he had asked to rate levels of pain. That they rated the same pain differently was reflected in relative brain activity. He concluded, "Showing that a person's report of how much something hurts matches their brain activity suggests that differences in pain perception are real, and doctors can trust what their patients tell them."[51] Consequently it is especially important that aspects of the patient's daily life and living conditions be taken into consideration. Pain is a whole-person event and specific to each individual person, making seeming tangents in a patient's description potentially valuable in determining the best possible treatment. That no one can perfectly know another's pain is indeed a problem. One's pain is finally hidden from others in a unique way; one cannot point to the experience as one might point to a bowl of kumquats and say, "See, that's what it is." Recognizing this difficulty is a critical part of the process of dealing with it.

It is a humbling recognition that demands attention to the variety of factors affecting a person's experience of pain. In his sustained meditation on how a person's cultural landscape and history determine her experience of pain, Morris promotes enriching the field of possibilities by drawing both from contemporary narratives of individuals' experiences and also from descriptions and interpretations that are a part of our largely forgotten or discounted literary heritage. Noting how difficult it is for a person in pain to find the words and then for others to listen, he explains the premise of his book as concerned with "achieving a new understanding of pain that allows us to recover the voices that mainstream medicine has rendered more or less unheard."[52] In so doing, he appeals both to the "neglected" voices of the patients themselves and to voices through literature — providing clarity, eloquence, and precision of description. Admitting that there is no way to communicate pain perfectly, Morris proposes that such attention "allow[s] us to examine various moments — specific historical junctures — when pain thrusts above the plane of silent, blind, unquestioned suffering in which it ordinarily lies concealed."[53] Closely reading ancient poetry from the biblical psalmists provides us an opportunity to witness such moments. The psalms express the difficulty of describing pain in ways that both raise questions about and proffer possibilities for managing pain.

As we have seen, the partner problem to that of describing pain is understanding it. The difficulty communicating one's own pain is matched by the challenge the other person faces in understanding it. However, the problem of understanding reaches much deeper, into questions of meaning itself. At the conclusion of her investigative and reflective book on pain, Jackson writes, "The exercise of investigating this subject has been similar to the needling challenge of a Buddhist koan. Pain's meaning is never separate from our experience of it, and yet to experience intense pain is to banish meaning."[54] This, then, is the central paradox of pain.

2

The Hermeneutics of Pain

*"A mind all logic is like a knife all blade. It makes
the hand bleed that uses it." —Babindranath Tagore*

Perhaps no other human experience so presses us for
explanation, so throws us back on metaphysical questions
of meaning and purpose as does pain. Furthermore, pain's
disruptive nature and the difficulties defining and communicating it call into question one's understanding of one's
very self. Pain challenges, chastises, and changes a person. Pain, with its attendant effects on every aspect of a
person's life, arrests that life. It evokes questions of meaning without providing clear answers or a new direction.
Pain calls into question earlier ideas about meaning and
demands their reassessment; it simultaneously both
denies, even destroys, meaning, and demands the (re)cre-
ation of meaning. Behind pain's many paradoxes lie the
questions: why? how long? what for? and even: who am
I? and what am I for?

We have inherited a modern understanding of pain that
is informed by the enthronement of science and reason, a
privileging that precludes understanding pain as anything
other than a physiological process. However, when pain is
understood as nothing other than impulses traveling along

nerve pathways, as nothing but a physiological phenomenon, questions of meaning are moot. Pain, according to
this model is then, by definition, meaningless. Yet, many
have observed that this sense of meaninglessness contributes to the agony of intractable pain. David Kahn and
Richard Steeves explain that painful suffering can be seen
"not as a meaning given to events that threaten personal
identity but as meaninglessness caused by that very
threat."[1] The sense of meaninglessness that so often comes
with chronic pain is ultimately bound up in the distinction
between body and mind. Morris explains that this was not
always so and need not continue to be. That is, our experience of pain is culturally based because it depends, in large
part, on how we interpret it. "Our biochemistry is inextricably bound up with the personal and cultural meanings
that we carve out of pain."[2] That pain presses us to seek
meaning is the felt pressure not only to survive, but to be
alive, whole persons integrated as body, mind, spirit, and
society. Meaning, then, and the process whereby a person
finds it must include all aspects of a person.

We are living in a period of great change in terms of our
understanding of pain. The model of pain as a purely
physiological phenomenon is undergoing a radical reshaping as more and more people experience pain that resists
treatment and find that the experience of chronic pain
affects them mentally, spiritually, and socially. Furthermore, the postmodern, postcolonial nature of our culture
stresses the polyvalent character of our experiences and
language. It undercuts the old hierarchies of power and
invites new voices and interpretations into discourse on
experience and truth. The recent and continuing boom
in multidisciplinary pain clinics attests both to the epidemic of pain and to the recognition of our need for new
ways of thinking about and dealing with it. We are

uniquely situated, then, to recognize how the search for meaning influences our experience of pain and plays a crucial role in the experience of pain itself.

The attempt to make meaning in and out of the experience of pain is an exercise in interpretation. However, in as much as interpretation is an intellectual pursuit, a person's interpretation of pain also and necessarily includes physiological, psychological, spiritual, and social influences/aspects; and any interpretation has equally wholistic consequences. Hermeneutics, the science of interpretation, asks about the manner in which people make sense of something. The exercise of meaning-making would seem to privilege cognitive processes. However, because a person's interpretation of pain is informed also by physiological, spiritual, and social experiences, meaning-making defies the reasonable conclusions of an intellectual exercise.

A hermeneutic of pain, an understanding of the process whereby a person interprets his or her pain, must take into account the wholistic nature of pain. An honest hermeneutic of pain is messy, and so the paradoxes of pain run even deeper. The conclusions of purely intellectual interpretations fall flat; making meaning in and out of pain defies conclusions that are not also necessarily process. "Answers" to questions about the genesis and purpose of pain fail to hold unless woven into them is the acknowledgment that they change with the dynamic and systemic nature of pain.

A hermeneutic of pain shows that interpretation is a process related as much by stories as by theories. Reading biblical psalms provides a lens through which we see how pain both presses people to ask questions of meaning and finally may defy answers to those questions. In doing so, however, the psalms suggest not that the answers are

wrong or have no value, but that the answers are bound
up in the experience of pain, which is itself dynamic. This
experience, then, trumps theories of its interpretation in
favor simply of telling the experience. The process of
telling integrates the experience of pain and ideas about
its meaning into the lived experience of a whole person.
Finally, that is, responses to questions about the meaning
of pain, its genesis and purpose, come rather to concern
meaning *in* pain, in the wrestling with pain and in
attempts to live through it.[3]

This paradoxical conclusion of a hermeneutic of pain—
that pain both demands and defies interpretation—is evident in the seemingly competing claims of two prominent
psychiatrists concerning meaning-making and pain. One,
Viktor Frankl, reflects the observation that pain demands
an account, some sense-making, and without that a person's pain is intolerable. The other, Arthur Kleinman,
reflects the observation that pain refuses such meaning-
making, and to attempt to impose meaning is to make a
person's pain intolerable. Frankl forged his theory in the
crucible of Auschwitz, where he determined that each life,
with all of its attendant suffering, must have meaning; and
that whatever meaning a life has is particular to each individual person. Frankl, a Viennese psychiatrist, wrote
Man's Search for Meaning, a small book that continues to
have great influence. His theory of logotherapy is based
on the supposition that "the striving to find a meaning in
one's life is the primary motivational force in man," and
the deepest meaning is the meaning of suffering.[4]

In apparent contrast to Frankl's enthronement of mean-
ing (yet also in response to the horror of the Holocaust),
Arthur Kleinman, a psychiatrist and anthropologist at
Harvard University, argues that attempts to establish

meaning actually compromise human development and self-realization. He writes, "The literary imagination's revulsion against, and the popular culture's reaction to, the bloody havoc of our century has challenged the dominion of meaning as inadequate, distorting, or even inhuman."[5] Kleinman challenges what he calls "a tyranny of meaning," an intellectual enterprise that fails to account properly for all of the variety of human experience and character. These two apparently incompatible ways of thinking about the hermeneutics of pain demonstrate another example of pain's paradoxical nature.

Although their conclusions appear to be polar opposites, Frankl and Kleinman are reconciled in the psalms. The experience of pain as expressed in the psalms both sanctions the importance of a search for meaning and demonstrates the manner in which determining a meaning yields simply to telling the experience and living in and through it. This transformation undercuts facile answers or one-dimensional, static conclusions about meaning. Instead, meaning is folded into the process of "getting on" with life in a manner that accounts for the real conditions of a person's multidimensional and dynamic nature. The candid and earnest wrestling with "why" questions are a part of that process, not an end to it. As the psalms both press for and posit meaning in the experience of pain, they also demonstrate that any meaning-making must be as dynamic as the experience itself. Such meaning-making is realized and expressed only in the telling. "The truth of stories is not only what was experienced, but equally what becomes experience in the telling and its reception."[6] Persistent and intractable pain presses us for meaning more than any other human experience, yet the meanings one may assign to it, like the pain itself, are dynamic and

resolved only in the living itself. Clarifying his criticism of
meaning-making, Kleinman observes a similar distinction
by defining problematic meaning-making as "a cognitive
response to the challenge of coherence."[7] That is, privileging the intellectual exercise over simply "inhabiting, acting
in, or wrestling with the world."[8] The psalms demonstrate
the tension between these enterprises—understanding
intellectually the experience of pain as meaningful, and
simply living meaningfully through (meaningless) pain.
The psalms do not discount the answers that people may
give to questions about the genesis and purpose of their
pain, but they relate them in the context of a personal cry.
The "answers" have a place, if only to be challenged and
sometimes abandoned by the experience and its expression. In an effort to understand this process, I describe
and discuss below some of the ways in which people interpret their pain. I then ask critically about the value and
problems with each one. Finally, I observe the manner in
which such interpretations may assume yet different
meaning and significance when woven into the lived experience of pain. And I observe how telling the experience is
itself a meaning-making exercise.

Where the Why Questions Lead

"A man is not destroyed by suffering, he is destroyed by
suffering without meaning," is the central tenet of Frankl's
teaching. Chronic and intractable pain challenges, compromises, and sometimes destroys a person's sense of self
and purpose. Why questions about the origins of pain and
the purpose for it are inseparable from questions about
who one is and for what. In other words, why questions
have implications for pathology; but they are also personal, with broad significance. Although they have to do
with the particular pathogenesis of disease and pain—

deterioration of vertebral disk, inflammation of meningeal structures of the brain, they also have to do with greater matters of purpose, suppositions about the world and one's place in it. Responses to such why questions are as varied as the experience of pain is. Yet they fall into four general categories: deserved pain, pain that improves a person, undeserved, and vicarious pain. Within each of these categories, interpretations are sensible in either religious or secular terms.

Pain as Deserved Punishment

Perhaps the most persistent interpretation of pain is as some kind of punishment. The etymology of our word *pain* itself reflects this—going back through Middle English to Old French *peine*, from Latin *poena*, and all the way back to Greek *poinê*, meaning simply "penalty." Understanding pain as deserved suffering may be the most common, and potentially problematic, of the general categories I cite. It can be simplistic and superficial or complicated and sophisticated. Whatever the case, at the heart of each such interpretation is the idea that one's pain is the just dessert for a particular wrongdoing. In religious terms, this manner of interpretation appears generally in the idea, "God is punishing me with this pain for some sin I have committed." In this case, God's character is understood as engaged in each individual human's life—God is just, and although powerful, God nevertheless allows for human freedom, an allowance that opens the door to misbehavior and the pain that follows. C. S. Lewis, writing in 1940, maintained that though it is a discomforting conclusion, pain is God's punishment, like it or not.[9] This model of interpretation presupposes that God is interested and involved in each person's life, engaged in yet not controlling. Consequently, when a person makes a bad decision out of his or her freedom to choose and act, God's justice demands punishment. The person's pain is a result of sin and a reflection of God's just action in that person's life.[10]

Another permutation of the religious interpretation of pain as deserved punishment is the idea that chronic and intractable pain reflects a failure of faith. We see this idea most frequently from the perspective of its implications, in the proliferation of "healing services" that aim to cure a person through fervent prayer and sacrifice. The logic of this particular interpretation dictates that if a person's condition does not improve, he or she or some member(s) of the group must be compromising, even sabotaging the healing process by insincerity of prayer or weakness of faith. Such an approach is founded in the presupposition that God desires all people to be well and with the right prayers and earnest belief, God will effect a cure.

The secular counterpart to the interpretation of pain as punishment is sensible simply by taking God out of the equation: we are naturally well beings; illness and pain are aberrations to our normal state of being. Yet people continuously make choices about their lives, on minute and grand levels, and each of these choices has implications, some of which include pain and suffering. The results are as myriad as the choices, with varying degrees of predictability. Easy examples come from the area of law and personal safety. Wearing a seatbelt is a legal requirement in many states, made so because of the clear correspondence between doing so and avoiding injury or even death in an accident. Choosing not to wear one's seatbelt is a crime (in religious language, a "sin"). The pain resulting from an accident is then understood as, in a sense, deserved. Other examples do not necessarily even depend on preexisting social rules. The area of preventive health is illustrative: exercise has been shown to reduce the risk of heart disease; the pain of a heart attack is understood as simply the penalty for eating too much unhealthy food and lounging on the couch every evening after a desk-job day. The person who chooses today to pick up the habit of smoking does so knowing that smoking carries enormous health risks; lung cancer, in this interpretive system, is considered the punitive result of the misbehavior of smoking. Steven Brena writes, "the principle of cosmic causation" provides an explanation, "where physical and mental calamities become the consequence of our present or past trespassing against natural or spiritual laws."[11]

Pain as Personal Improvement

The interpretation of pain as personal improvement considers pain as a blessing in disguise — bane that with the right attitude becomes boon. The religious form of this interpretation shares with that of pain-as-deserved-punishment the idea that God is just and powerful and immediately involved in each person's life. It also may interpret pain as punishment but in a corrective rather than payment-of-debts manner. That is, to this way of thinking, although pain is associated with wrongdoing, it is simply a means to the greater end by instruction through correction. The idea that God uses pain to improve a person frequently gives rise to the assertion that God teaches by means of pain. An early champion of this interpretation is the second-century theologian, Irenaeus, who argued, "Suffering is understood both as inevitable — because of human imperfection — and as pedagogical and salutary. It is through suffering that one grows closer to the ideal for which one was created; suffering is part of the perfecting process."[12]

One form of the secular counterpart to this interpretation of pain as personal improvement emerges as the belief that pain leads people to reconsider their priorities. Betty Ferrell observes, "Outcomes of life reappraisal include an increased appreciation for human relationships, greater self-understanding, and stronger positive attitudes regarding life."[13] Pain directs a person to focus on "what really matters." Comparing his experiences as a medical doctor in the United States, Great Britain, and India, Paul Brand, author of *Pain: The Gift Nobody Wants*, observes that despite generally worse conditions and specifically untreated pain, poor Indians seemed happier than the wealthy Americans and English who had access to a wide variety of pain-relieving drugs and therapies.[14] Another form of the interpretation of pain as personal improvement is echoed in Nietzche's oft-repeated maxim, "what does not kill you makes you stronger." According to this thinking, one's present pain will effect greater resilience, even ability, in that person in the future. "No pain, no gain," as the saying goes. Yet another form of this interpretation is that the pain is a necessary part of treatment that will cure an underlying condition. For example, the chemotherapy and radiation that cancer patients undergo can be terribly painful, yet it is designed to arrest and/or reverse the cancer, thereby enabling remission and/or recovery.

Pain as Undeserved Suffering

The interpretation of pain as undeserved suffering reflects a manner of making meaning out of the lack of meaning. In religious terms, God does not will that innocent people suffer, but the nature of the world is such that pain is inevitable and God-given freedoms preclude God's direct intervention to spare undeserving people unnecessary pain. Another translation of this interpretation admits ignorance of God's intentions and plans. God's ways are mysterious, and so we cannot know how and why people suffer pain. One can see how easily this interpretation bends to the other two. Not knowing the whole story leaves open the possibility that a person has unwittingly done something to deserve the pain and/or that God is working in seemingly undeserved pain to effect a greater purpose.

Another way to think about pain that is undeserved is to distinguish between the innocence of an individual in the context of the guilt of a group. "Collective punishment" includes the undeserving innocents in its accounting of the guilty. Although many associate such thinking with the Old Testament, and indeed it is reflected there (e.g. Exodus 34:7 describes God as one who holds children accountable "to the third and fourth generations" for the sins of their progenitors), it is also challenged within Old Testament texts explicitly (e.g. we read in Ezekiel 18:4, "only the person who sins shall die") and implicitly (e.g. in the story of Abraham's bargaining with God to consider sparing Sodom rather than destroying righteous individuals along with the city's sinful majority [Genesis 18]).

A purely secular understanding of undeserved pain allows little discussion: that's just the way it is; life's unfair; pain happens. In an essay that begins, "He has seen but half the universe who has never been Shewn the house of Pain," R. W. Emerson expresses such a perspective. However, this nineteenth-century American transcendentalist optimistically considers that the intellect affords a person the emotional distance that enables him or her to use the pain for the purpose of art. He writes, "The bitterest tragic element in life to be derived from an intellectual source is the belief in a brute Fate or Destiny," and continues, "But this terror [. . .] disappears with civilization. [. . .] The intellect is a consoler, which delights in detach-

ing or putting an interval between a man and his fortune,
and so converts the sufferer into a spectator and his pain
into poetry."[15]

There is also a secular counterpart to the biblical notion
of collective punishment. Interpreting an individual's
undeserved pain as an effect of a group's misdeeds is evident in many contemporary interpretations of national
and global ills. The problem of air pollution, for example,
with its attendant afflictions of skin and lung cancers,
asthma, and eye irritations can be understood as collective
punishment for the failure to take seriously the effects of
our choices and behavior on the environment on which we
depend. Again, while the painful conditions are experienced on an individual level, they are the product of insti-
tutional and national misdeeds—"the group," in other
words. Yet within the suffering group are individuals who
have worked to avoid the problem of air pollution in the
first place and often precisely in order to avoid its attendant pains.

Pain Suffered on account of Others

The interpretation of pain suffered on account of others
seems as old as religion itself. Generally speaking, it is sac-
rificial: the assumption of pain by a person or group as a
substitute for or redemption of others. The "suffering servant" in the book of Isaiah is described as taking on the
pain and humiliation that the servant's group deserved to
suffer on account of their sins. In doing so, the servant
both identifies with the group and is distinguished from
them. The servant suffers *their* pain so that they might be
reconciled to God and so be spared the punishment that
was their due. There are many other examples of such fig-
ures in the Hebrew Bible, but it is Isaiah's suffering servant that provides the template for the early Christian

community's understanding of the person and role of Jesus.

Today some people interpret their pain in such a manner, but in religious terms it appears most frequently in the sense of sharing in God's own suffering. This is especially common among Christians who understand the pain of a crucified Jesus as ongoing among the community of his followers continuing what they understand to be his work, begun and passed along to them. To Christians who understand their pain as sharing in the suffering of Christ, Roman Catholic priest and hospital chaplain Robert Smith warns, "this is a mysterious and extremely delicate understanding of suffering. It should never be imposed on someone else." He cautions that such an interpretation must be made out of love, and be "filled with the wisdom of experience and compassion" and avoid self-aggrandizement.[16]

In secular terms, pain suffered on account of others is the acceptance of pain so that others avoid or are relieved of it. Emmanuel Levinas, who judges pain to be a kind of evil, nevertheless comments on its ability to effect good when interpreted as undertaken for the benefit of someone else. He observes first, "The evil which rends the humanity of a suffering person, overwhelms his humanity otherwise than non-freedom overwhelms it. [. . .] The evil of pain, the harm itself, is the [. . .] most profound articulation of absurdity."[17] But he continues by noting that suffering on account of the suffering of another assumes meaning, even in its uselessness, and he accords it a great value. Taking this even further, he argues that such suffering for the Other (on account of the other's suffering) is actually obligatory.[18]

Viktor Frankl tells the story of an elderly physician who came to him for psychotherapy because of unresolved grief and depression following his wife's death. Frankl listened to the man's complaint, and instead of answering, responded with the question of how things might have been if the man had died before his wife did. "'Oh,' he said, 'for her this would have been terrible; how she would have suffered!'"[19] Thinking about his situation in this way gave the man a sense of meaning for and in his pain that transformed it from intolerable to tolerable. Similarly, the pain of injuries sustained from saving the life of another may be tolerable whereas the pain from similar injuries sustained from an accident or assault may be intolerable.

Interrogating Interpretations

Although each of these categories of interpretation are sensible, and it is possible to determine how a person might arrive at each, there are problems with each of them, too. For example, interpreting pain as deserved punishment is entirely inappropriate in some cases. People who suffered brutal abuse as children frequently bring feelings of guilt and shame into their adult years, having incorporated ideas that they deserved the pain of their abuse. However, there are also cases wherein an interpretation of pain as deserved punishment is not so easily dismissed. It may well satisfy a person's sense of his or her pain in a way that gives it meaning and suggests a manner of end—when the punishment is satisfied. Finding a sense for the pain, a meaning for its origin and a meaning for what it will accomplish may give the sufferer comfort. Whatever the case, finally it is "cold comfort," as Episcopal priest and author Frederick Schmidt observes.[20] As the pain continues unremittingly, a person is undone; and such interpretations become destructive and dehumanizing, sometimes also creating conditions of greater pain for others. Furthermore, such interpretations have problematic and ultimately unsatisfactory theological implications. Ideas of God purely as judge, demanding right behavior and punishing for wrong, are dangerously narrow and finally unbiblical. Not only is the principle of God consistently punishing wrongdoing and rewarding the right untenable, insofar as many of those who do wrong suffer no ill effects and vice versa, but also such ideas of God as absolute judge discount the ability of God to exercise mercy and grace, attributes that get a good deal of attention in biblical texts.

The interpretation of pain as undeserved suffering is also both sensible and problematic. It avoids some of the problematic implications of the above two categories of interpretation but it introduces others. It avoids the self-flagellation that thinking of pain as just punishment can produce, and it avoids the pious, martyr perspective that understanding one's pain as self-improvement may elicit. Simply to note that pain does not distinguish between "good" and "bad" people, that it happens without concern for the balance of justice, is realistic; and in its honesty, such an interpretation may be comforting to those in pain. It may relieve a person both of the agonizing quest to determine what he or she did wrong to elicit such pain and of the despair and self-loathing that attend assumptions about pain as somehow deserved.

However, simply determining that one's pain is undeserved does not provide lasting comfort. It finally is not a meaning, and "Any meaning of illness is better than none," the dying Anatole Broyard observed.[21] Although it derives from a valuable sense of self-worth and an honest inability to find good reason for chronic pain, it may leave a person disillusioned and effectively paralyzed. There is nothing left for a person to do with this interpretation, no teleology, no purpose for the pain. Consequently, as the pain continues, a person who ascribes to such an interpretation cannot help but feel demoralized and depressed. Questions about what to *do* with the pain remain, as do questions about a person's identity and purpose in the context of chronic and intractable pain.

The interpretation of pain as undeserved is categorically different from the first two interpretations because of its implications for understanding the character and role of God, or natural conditions and processes. One way that the interpretation of pain as undeserved appears in religious terms allows little discussion. God is capricious and/or unjust and the result is that some people suffer great pain for no good reason. Although it may be interpreted as punishment, and understood as such, the pain is nevertheless considered unequal or unrelated to the choices and behavior of the person (or group) in pain. One example is the infant badly injured at birth and looking forward to a life filled with surgeries and disabilities. Evaluated theologically, such cases suggest either that God is disinterested in, absent from, or unable to act in human affairs or that God is malicious, capricious, and/or sadistic. Some argue that a God under whose watch undeserved pain happens cannot be all-powerful and just (consequently, not worth the title "God"). W. E. B. DuBois, wrestled with this in his antiphonal poem "A Litany of Atlanta," composed after the September 22, 1906 race riot that killed twenty-four African-Americans. He writes, "Is this Thy Justice, O Father, that guile be easier than innocence and the innocent crucified for the guilt of the untouched guilty? *Justice, O Judge of men!*"

The atheist Ivan, in Fyodor Dostoevsky's *Brothers Karamazov*, poignantly challenges his Christian brother, Alyosha, regarding the idea that one person's undeserved pain is the result of God punishing the group's sins. Ivan says of the suffering of innocent children, "If they, too, suffer horribly on earth, they must suffer for their fathers' sins, they must be punished for their fathers, who have eaten the apple; but that reasoning is of the other world and is incomprehensible for the heart of man here on the earth. The innocent must not suffer for another's sins, and especially such innocents!"[22] Ivan also addresses the suffering of the innocent one at the hands of another whose torturing is itself the crime. In such a case, the innocent's suffering is not payment for the punishment of another's crime but is (only) the direct effect of that crime. He says, "Those tears are unatoned for. They must be atoned for, or there can be no harmony. But how? How are you going to atone for them? Is it possible? By their being avenged? But what do I care for avenging them? What do I care for a hell for oppressors? What good can hell do, since those children have already been tortured?"[23]

Such questions imply also that interpreting pain as undeserved without using religious terminology is no more satisfying. Simply stating that sometimes pain happens is hardly to give the pain meaning or purpose. Furthermore, in the case of the pain suffered by an individual on account of the abuse of another, punishment and/or atonement of the criminal does not erase the effect of his or her crime on the victim. The Korean concept of *han* gives a name to the pain of the abuser's victim. It is a particularly problematic pain that can cycle back into new abuses as the victim, trying to come to terms with his or her pain, may actually become the perpetrator.[24]

As is true with interpretations of pain as deserved and as undeserved, the interpretation of pain as personal improvement makes sense and so has a place in certain experiences of pain, but it also poses some practical and theological problems. A person may acknowledge certain self-destructive or socially problematic behaviors when faced with an intractable pain. The pain, then, either directly prohibits continuing to engage in such behaviors or indirectly prompts him or her to correct the behavior. Such an interpretation of pain is related to the potential of pain to focus a person on "what really matters," enabling him or her to appreciate relationships and simple things in and about life that also imbue meaning and purpose in that life. However, such an interpretation can also become destructive in its potential for masochism and the development of a martyr complex. Furthermore, although pain may indeed focus a person in ways that yield life-affirming benefits, most people discover that it is impossible to sustain such an attitude with pain that is chronic and intractable. In those times, such an interpretation may yield to despair and self-disgust as the person finds himself or herself unable even to appreciate the "good things." This interpretation also has problematic theological implications—that God is sadistic, visiting pain on people in order to teach them to love life and appreciate the world and each other. Again, biblical texts undermine such an interpretation as they portray a God who employs a number of other, less toxic, techniques to accomplish such lofty goals.

That most interpretations of pain fall into one or another of the above described categories attests to the validity of these interpretations. In other words, there is something about each one that seems true to individuals' experiences of pain. That there are several different categories, and many different interpretations, attests to the diversity not only of the experience of pain but also of the meanings people make out of pain. No one interpretation is satisfactory in every case. Indeed, a hermeneutic of pain must account for the fact that each person's meaning-making is influenced not only by a number of factors — physiological, psychological, spiritual, and social/cultural, but also that there is great diversity within the factors. In the face of the reality that each of these interpretations has something to commend it but that none of them are finally satisfactory, we witness the paradox of the importance of making meaning out of pain (Frankl's position) and the danger of doing so (Kleinman's position). The attempt to find meaning in the experience of pain is important and valuable, but no conclusion proffers itself as finally satisfying the why questions of pain's genesis and purpose. Furthermore, each kind of interpretation has the potential for great harm, and not only to the individual person suffering chronic and intractable pain.

Integrating Interpretations

Narrative bridges the divide and reconciles these competing truths about the place of meaning-making in the experience of pain. In telling, we find the dynamism that characterizes pain and that is lacking in any fixed interpretation. In telling, we find both a place for these interpretations and a means of living in and through them to seek the reintegration of a person composed of and consistently influenced by body, mind, spirit, and community. This is not to say that it is necessary for each individual to create an autobiography. Rather, it is to appreciate that in narrative, one's own or another's, we find a candor that is lacking in fixed interpretations and prescribed therapies.[25] In his popular book, *When Bad Things Happen to Good People*, Harold Kushner reflects on the biblical story of Job, a faultless man who nevertheless suffers enormously. Kushner observes that when Job's three friends attempt to find meaning for his suffering, they wrongly interpret Job's "why me?" as a question seeking a theological answer rather than simply a cry of pain. "What Job needed from his friends [. . .] was not theology, but sympathy."[26] Before they spoke, Kushner writes, the friends did two things right: they came to be with Job, and they listened to him.

The psalms model the importance of seeking and determining meaning for the experience of pain, but they do so in the context of a process. There is a place for a person to claim understanding for the genesis and purpose of his or her pain; but if such interpretations become fixed and determinative, they open the door to the problems cited above. Stasis renders them untrue and risks contributing further to the disintegration of the pained person. "In the going, I'm already there."[27] The psalms demonstrate the place for and through such interpretations in shifting voices and tones as the psalmists seek not only to understand their experiences of pain but also simply to live in and through them.

While philosophers and theologians bend their minds to the challenges of defining and describing the genesis and purpose of pain and the theological implications for such interpretations, the psalms show both the power of different interpretations and that those interpretations change and/or are rendered moot simply by the experience and expression of pain. Interpretations such as we considered above have an important place in the sense-making that pain demands, but they are not finally the only or even most critical part of the process of reintegrating the self. There are problems with each seeming solution, problems that may finally interfere with a person's healing reintegration. The psalms model the movement of narrative, a self-story that accommodates interpretation into expression in a manner that may not finally "add up" to a neat formula in answer to the why questions of pain's genesis and purpose. Considering the psalms in light of the problems of pain shows that the search for sense in and of the experience is indeed important, but so is figuring out simply how to get along, as they wrestle with, complain about, grieve, and delight in the myriad aspects of life. Each of the four categories of interpretation is evident in the psalms, in one way or another, but none of the psalms proposes that its particular interpretation is finally satisfactory. Instead, each psalm models the dynamism of the experience of pain and the consequently necessary dynamism of thinking about and dealing with it. Although they validate the search for meaning that pain requires of sufferers, they eschew the idea that meaning finally fully answers the experience of pain.

The psalms do not always model a fully reintegrated person and they are no more prescriptive than they are systematically theological. Just as we cannot turn to them for a sophisticated and scientific description of who and how God is, neither can we simply apply them to the experience of pain for answers and relief. However, the psalms do represent an honest cry out of pain, the search for meaning and "trying on" interpretations, and the expression of pain as a dynamic experience with implications for the sufferer that are systemic. In the process, the psalmists weave all aspects of their whole persons into an audible cry that draws hearers, even all of these centuries later, into the sufferer's community.

The metaphysical questions that pain evokes reveal the inseparability of body, mind, and spirit, disclosing the "Myth of Two Pains," as Morris calls our misleading tendency to talk about physical versus mental pain. While the meaning-destroying power of pain fractures the self into pieces such as body, mind, and spirit (and further into pieces of the pieces) and the individual from his or her greater community, the metaphysical questions it evokes invite the sufferer to seek ways to reintegrate the self. Just as pain's relation to meaning underlies the paradox of pain as simultaneously physical and mental, so it underlies the paradox of pain as simultaneously particular and universal, both impossible to tell and demanding that one do so. Indeed, while the quest of reintegration is, by definition, a personal and individualistic journey, it is paradoxically also social—bound by culture, based in narrative, and engaging others. The telling of pain that we witness in the psalms represents an attempt to make sense of the experience as it bears on the whole person, physically, psychologically, spiritually, and socially. Such telling presumes a listener and so creates a social relationship. We become a part of that relationship by reading the dynamic experience of pain, complaint, meaning-making, grief, and sometimes relief. Furthermore, that the psalms are all defined by address to God quietly, yet unfailingly, suggests that this God is a God of relationship, promoting the process of being with and for others, and leaving no one alone in his or her pain.

3

Pain and the Psalms,
Beyond the Medicine Cabinet

✒

"Who shall ascend into the hill of the Lord? Or who shall stand in his holy place? There is no one but us. There is no one to send, nor a clean hand, nor a pure heart on the face of the earth, nor in the earth, but only us." —Annie Dillard

In the chapters that follow, I look closely at six psalms, asking not only what they say but also how they demonstrate and/or challenge some of what we have observed about the experience and expression of pain in general. In so doing, I aim to prepare readers to understand and appreciate what the psalms might offer for how we understand and manage different aspects of the pain experience. I do not propose that there is a one-to-one correspondence between the psalms and pain relief, or that there are cures hidden or encoded within the text. To approach the psalms looking for application like pharmaceuticals, surgery, or physical therapy is to reduce them to little more than alternatives within the medicine cabinet of pain-relievers. Allowing our inquiry a category different from such techniques is not to deny the importance of pharmaceutical and medical procedures but is simply to allow for a different way of thinking about pain, its experience and management.

Lately, there has been an explosion of interest in the relationship between religion and health, as studies claiming that religiously active people tend to be healthier and live longer than others gain in popularity. Similarly, there has been increased interest in the healing effects of prayer, leading some to consider the psalms as little more than prayers that God likes and so will respond to favorably.[1] As with so much of life and so many of the biblical texts, it is more complicated than that. I hope that closely reading these six psalms and discussing particular aspects of them will enrich our ways of thinking about pain and how to live fully through it. The process of listening to these ancient poems and engaging them with questions and reflection enables ways of thinking about and dealing with one's own pain and the pain of others that facilitate the integration of fractured selves and so a return to the wholeness/holiness of a healthy life.

The psalms bear testimony to processes of telling pain, interpreting, and seeking relief from it; consequently, readers of these texts become witnesses to the personal narratives of people in pain. The usefulness of closely reading these particular psalms, therefore, is not limited to those in pain or to those (Jews and Christians) for whom the texts are considered authoritative. I hope this reading of particular psalms is sensible not only to those who believe the Bible to be "Word of God," but also to others willing to listen to the psalmist's cry and participate in his or her struggle to make sense of and live through pain. I hope that attending to the texts as we do here sensitizes caregivers, medical and otherwise, to the religious beliefs and perspectives that affect their patients' understanding and management of pain; but I also hope that it is useful, no matter what is the reader's religious background, to those who are in pain and to those who care for persons in pain. The importance of listening to such psalms has a reach beyond Judaism and Christianity. It is to participate in the process of meaning-making and the quest to reintegrate a fractured self that form the basis of healing. There is no neat lesson here, reducible to an applicable formula. There is instead an invitation to experience and question, to participate in a process that accounts for the reality of sickness and death and seeks a health that is wholeness/holiness in person and community, even through pain. In this brief introduction to the six chapters concerning individual psalms, I identify several reasons why the psalms might be considered a resource for pain management today, include a warning about the dangers that readers face in dealing with ancient religious texts, and explain what it is about these six psalms in particular that commends them for consideration here.

The Significance of Ancient Psalms for Today's Pain

The book of Psalms is appropriate for consideration in the context of contemporary questions about pain management for several reasons, which I list in this paragraph and develop more fully below. One, biblical texts continue to inform our culture; and two, Psalms is unique among biblical books for its personal tone. Three, besides reflecting the radically subjective nature of pain, the psalms reflect pain's dynamic character, ever-changing in experience, interpretation, and understanding. Furthermore, the psalms presume that a healthy person is naturally whole — not separable into what we call physical, mental, and spiritual aspects; and they presume that that wholeness is defined also by proper integration of the individual in the greater society. Finally, the psalms require an audience. The psalmist speaks and readers listen. In that speaking and listening is an activity crucial to the reintegration of an individual as self and member of the greater community.

It is the thesis of David Morris's book *The Culture of Pain* that "the experience of pain is decisively shaped or modified by individual human minds and by specific human cultures."[2] I agree with him that our literary heritage is a fundamental part of our culture. However, while Morris laments the loss of historical literacy, of an awareness and engagement among people today with the rich resources "from Homer to Beckett," we can appreciate the continued popularity of the Bible. That is not to say that people have been unflaggingly well educated about the Bible, its history, literature, and theology; but we can say that it has been a living text with considerable influence through the centuries and into today. It has been interpreted and (re)interpreted famously in art such as Michelangelo's sculpture of David, Leonardo DaVinci's painting of the Last Supper, the music of G. F. Handel's "Messiah," and the poetry of John Milton's "Paradise Lost." The Bible's Exodus provided a rich metaphor for the antebellum South, described as a kind of Egypt by African-American slaves. Biblical stories and poetry have been a foundation and inspiration for such influential literature as Herman Melville's *Moby Dick*, Toni Morrison's *Song of Solomon*, and William Faulkner's *Absalom! Absalom!* In his first presidential address to the nation after the disaster of September 11, 2001, George W. Bush appealed to Psalm 23. Sometimes without our recognition and regardless of our faith perspective; the Bible informs and influences our greater worldview. The psalms are part of our cultural make-up and a rich inheritance with which to engage today.

Further commending them for consideration here, the psalms are highly subjective, indeed personal, a characteristic (also of pain) that is unique among biblical texts. No other book of the Bible is so composed of people's words to God out of their particularly human experiences. Its poetry reflects the wide range of such experiences — philosophizing, questioning, celebrating, raging, grieving, reminiscing, and giving thanks. Among them, however, the most common are psalms that express more bleak human thoughts and emotions such as grief, anger, despair, fear, and loneliness. The terminology biblical scholars use for a psalm dominated by such expressions is "lament." While other kinds of psalms lend themselves to analysis by literary structure and organization, the laments frequently do not — how like pain. Claus Westermann, a leading voice in Psalms research, observed, "[Lament psalms] do not follow a set pattern, rather the order and succession of motifs is quite free and very variable. All they have in common is that the principal motifs are the same and that they all describe a movement though not always in the same way, which develops from the lament."[3]

Indeed, this dynamism is yet another justification for applying psalms to inquiry in the area of pain management. Just as the experience of pain is ever-changing, readers witness development in each psalmists' reasoning and expression of pain. While psalms of lament describe an unenviable condition of the psalmist, they do not stop there. Instead, we witness the psalmist changing in and through the experience. However, there is no specific pattern of movement that each psalmist follows; rather, like the individual nature of the experience of pain, different psalms manage the problem and its attendant issues differently. Consequently, they demonstrate processes of expressing and understanding pain that are meaningful both for those who are in pain and for those who care for them. That is, these psalms provide a vocabulary and language for expressing pain, a grammar of pain, which continues to resonate for people struggling with difficulties understanding and describing their particular experiences of suffering.

A critical characteristic of this "grammar of pain" is its inclusion of all aspects of the self. The psalmists seem less interested in describing the specific nature of physical pain than they do in expressing the effects of such suffering. That is, psalmic descriptions of pain are rarely the sort of particular explanations that would aid in making a medical diagnosis but are rather exclamations out of pain that describe the overall effect and toll such suffering exacts. Indeed, although I began my research with a focus on physical pain, I found that the psalms defy such clear distinctions; the psalms' descriptions of suffering blur the boundaries between physical, psychological, spiritual, and social pain. Hints and descriptions of physical pain do not stand alone or serve as the subjects of greater description and elaboration. Instead, they are interwoven with expressions of the psalmist's emotional and spiritual experiences.

Striking among these individualized expressions is the importance the psalmist accords to his or her community. That is, nearly all psalms that have something to do with pain also say something about the psalmist's social condition. There is a profound social dimension inherent in the psalmists' telling. This has important implications for pain management today, as suggested by Naomi Eisenberger's recent neuroimaging study demonstrating a link in the brain between social rejection and the experience of (physical) pain. Her research has been popularly described as demonstrating a broken heart. Eisenberger explains, "evidence suggests that some of the same neural machinery recruited in the experience of physical pain may also be involved in the experience of pain associated with social separation or rejection."[4] The psalmists describe such a relationship, thereby extending their "wholistic" reach beyond the individual, composed of interwoven aspects, to include an understanding of the individual as inextricably bound up in the whole of the greater social group.

Consequently, it may not be surprising to note that another way in which the psalms are relevant in the search to manage pain is that they demand to be heard. That is, their inclusion in the Bible, poignantly personal tone, and expression of a dynamic experience involving the whole self and the whole self in community requires attention. They demand of readers a hearing, just as does a person in pain, seeking to incorporate his or her experience of pain into the whole of a life. On the other hand, they also give voice to bodies and show solidarity to or with others in pain.[5] The telling and hearing are crucial as a person experiences and creates community in telling his or her pain for personal relief and shares his or her pain for others' relief. The psalms do not give us an answer to the question of how to cure pain. They demonstrate earnest attempts to manage it within a whole life, portraying the very real experience of pain and telling in various ways the effects of that experience. In the telling and attendant meaning-making, they testify to a timeless human quest for wholeness/holiness/health in an imperfect world and with finite lives. Therefore, they commend themselves as relevant among contemporary efforts to alleviate pain, both one's own and that of others. The psalms are appropriate for a contemporary inquiry of pain because they are a part of our culture, subjective, dynamic, and wholistic, concerning both self and society, and to read them is to be a witness to another's testimony of life experience.

Dangers of an Easy (Re)Application of Psalms

Despite the currency that biblical texts continue to have in our culture, there are some real difficulties in looking to psalms for application today. For one thing, they are far distant from us in time and space. Their compositions date somewhere between 2,300 to 3,000 or more years ago, and so the psalms derive from and reflect periods of time very different from our own. Furthermore, the sites of their composition span an ancient Near-Middle East quite different in landscape from today's Near-Middle East (and quite different from the locales of many reading this book), infusing the poetry with a foreignness that can complicate our understanding of them. Finally, despite the continuing life of these ancient texts in today's religious traditions and culture in general, they also reflect and grow out of theological and cultural assumptions and traditions that are in many ways different from our own.

In an attempt to bridge this gap, a dizzying amount of research has been done on the psalms, spanning a wide range of inquiry including the identification of historical contexts, literary forms, and theological themes. In the course of such study, a few general things have become apparent, and they may be summed up with two words: various and unknown. That is, there is great variety among the psalms and there continues to be much that we do not know about them. For example, apart from knowing that they come from a variety of circumstances, it is not possible to place most psalms definitively in a particular, original, historical and social setting. One effect of this is that the psalms have a timelessness, defying exclusive identification with a specific event and/or use. Similarly, the psalms represent a variety of literary types, again reflecting the breadth of human experience and expression. Furthermore, there is no systematic theology that one can mine from the book of Psalms. That is, the psalms do not together portray one image of God that conforms to a particular profile or formula. Together, the psalms suggest that God looks like a person, yet cannot be personified; God is angry and punishing, yet calm and comforting; God is immediate, yet remote; personable, yet mysterious; in short, paradoxical.

In a recent work, biblical scholar Jerome Creach proposed that the image of God as refuge might embrace the variety of images and so provide consistency throughout the psalms;[6] but not all descriptions of God conform to this idea. Building on Creach's work, William Brown proposed a twofold theological understanding that includes the notion of "way" alongside that of God as refuge. He observes the importance that the psalmists give to Torah, specifically obedience to Torah—serious application of the instruction of God, as the means to living a good life.[7] Indeed, despite their variety, nearly all of the lament psalms include reference to either the psalmist's or others' failure to know and observe Torah as contributing to the pain expressed. Consequently, many people today assume that the Bible blames the sufferer for his or her pain: the sufferer has done something to deserve this punishment from God. This is not without support in the biblical texts, but it requires a more nuanced understanding that takes into account both the variety of images of God and the importance biblical texts accord God's instruction to human beings. *Torah*, as described and portrayed in biblical texts, is less the kind of oppressive legal strictures and mandates, which the term "God's law" connotes, than a gift of divine instruction that facilitates living a full and satisfying life. These interpretations bear consideration in our study of pain in the psalms where we will see them confirmed . . . and challenged, with important implications for how the psalms might be instructive and useful to people in pain and to those who care for them.

In the process of asking about such application of the psalms, it is crucial to avoid a contemporary desire to look to them to make us better. In contrast to the cultural and historical context of the authors of these biblical poems, we live in an individualistic, market-driven culture, which emphasizes feel-good youth and a sense that everyone deserves health and wealth, defined by no suffering and lots of money. While the psalms certainly reflect individual voices telling of the timeless human desire to avoid or at least minimize suffering and sometimes of material satisfaction, they are not founded or primarily focused on such. Their perspective is theological and practical as they wrestle differently with how to live fully in the midst of suffering and in the midst of a greater community. In short, they demonstrate an effort to live, in all states of health and illness, with integrity as an individual within a social group. It is this integrity that is at the foundation of health and wealth and that accounts for the crucial nature of relationships—to God, others, and the world around, in defining a good life. Reintegrating a self fractured by pain involves a process of identifying, understanding, and describing the experience in an effort to live fully through the pain. This is not a linear process from fracture to mending and so to completion. Developing a narrative of one's life that includes the experience of pain requires both telling and listening in a constant back-and-forth. It is both to articulate one's experience and interpretation and to participate in others' articulation of their own in a continuous process. In short, care must be taken in looking to psalms for contemporary relevance because they reflect conditions and presumptions different from ours. They are distant from us in time and place, do not present a systematic theology, and they suggest that pain management is more a process of self and social integration than a function of identifying and applying a particular cure.

Why These Six Psalms in Particular

To appreciate what the psalms offer requires close reading, a careful listening to and engagement with them. However, the number relevant for the question of pain is great. Of the 150 psalms within the book of Psalms, at least thirty deal specifically with pain. They include 6, 9, 22, 25, 31, 32, 38, 39, 40, 41, 42, 44, 55, 69, 73, 77, 88, 102, 103, 107, 109, 116, 118, 119, 130, 142, 143, 145, 146, and 147. Psalms 7, 10, 13, 18, 30, 34, 35, 56, 57, 59, 63, 70, 71, 72, 120, and 130 also make reference to pain, though in some cases obliquely. The six psalms (6, 22, 38, 69, 88, and 102) that I have chosen to read closely reflect and deal powerfully with the experience of pain, and they do so in quite different ways.

When I set about to determine the kinds of pain that the psalmists suffer, I discovered that they seldom spelled it out. The terms that appear most frequently to describe pain are the most general – *'oni* which translates as "affliction, misery, poverty" and *tsarah* which translates as "distress, anxiety, need." By contrast, the most specific conditions described in "plain speech" are the most rare. One verse tells of festering wounds (38:5) and another of disjointed bones (22:14), yet both could finally be meant metaphorically after all. Many descriptions tell of suffering by reference both to pain's specific effects, for example an inability to see, speak, hear, eat, and/or sleep, and to its general effects such as losing strength and wholeness, and feeling on the verge of death. There are numerous references to weariness, the exhaustion of dealing with persistent pain. Of these, many tell of wasting away, drying up, being trampled or bowed down. The psalmists make frequent use of metaphors and similes to produce evocative images such as a heart melting like wax (22:14), the inability to secure firm footing (38:17; 40:2; 69:2, 14), feeling bound up or imprisoned (e.g. 25:15; 31:4; 116:16), and the overwhelming sensation of drowning (42:7; 69:1, 2, 14, 15; 88:7, 16-17). In *The Body in Pain*, Elaine Scarry proposes that pain defies communication in its world-unmaking quality (but that it lies behind every act of creation). Although the depth of despair expressed by several psalms seems to confirm her impression, the psalms also challenge this perspective concerning the articulation of pain. They are expressions of pain. Although they decline to describe details of physical pain, they demonstrate the human struggle to communicate the nature of anguish, to identify its sources, to describe its effects, and to secure relief.

Most psalms associate the speaker's pain with a social situation. Although the experience of pain is profoundly individual, the sufferer is part of a greater community that for better or worse informs and affects him or her. Nearly all psalms having to do with pain identify unnamed enemies as a (but not always *the*) source of suffering or pain. The only exceptions are Psalms 103 and 107, not spoken out of pain but rather praising God's forgiveness/healing; Psalm 116, also not spoken out of pain but remembering God's saving action; and Psalm 130, which may not actually have any reference to physical pain. "The depths" mentioned there may not be spatial, but rather psychological or spiritual. Psalms 145, 146, and 147 praise God for general acts of salvation in third person descriptions. Psalm 39 might be added to this group; however, it associates the psalmist's pain with the ignorance of others and anticipates their scorn. With the possible exception of Psalm 39, all psalms spoken out of pain include a social element, and frequently it is critical in tone, citing either others' actively contributing to the psalmist's pain or their failure to relieve it.

Although close readings reveal how complicated and multifaceted are the psalmists' experiences, interpretation, and management of pain, each psalm emphasizes something identifiably distinct. Psalm 6 demonstrates a process of moving pain out of the center of the psalmist's life and thought. Psalm 22 tells of the pain of profound loneliness/abandonment, then of joy in and thanks for a new integration with a community of others. Psalm 38 reflects the sense of pain as the just punishment of God, yet following repentance, looks to God for help. The poet of Psalm 69 is especially concerned with reasons for the pain. The darkest of all, Psalm 88, expresses despair and exhaustion with a sense of abandonment from God who exacerbates the pain. The finitude of a person's life in comparison to an eternal God is at the heart of Psalm 102, which moves from despair at such condition to appreciation of it.

In the process of listening to these psalms and reflecting on their assumptions, perspectives, questions, and conclusions, we participate as witnesses in the testimony of pain. We become active partners in the meaning-making of selves seeking repair. Experiencing the permeability of boundaries between aspects of the self and between the self and others, we become better able to reintegrate the self (our own and that of others) both as an individual whole and within the greater social whole. The psalms do not tell us how to live through pain; they invite active participation in the process itself.

Why This Particular (Noncanonical) Order of the Psalms

I have not followed the ordering of psalms as they appear in the Bible. Their order here reflects, instead, the particular topic of this book. The book of Psalms is not organized around the issue of pain, neither is its order random. However, the characteristic of psalms as individual literary units allows us to discuss them in an order that draws attention generally to the dynamic experience of pain. This is not to say that the context of individual psalms within the greater book (their situation vis-à-vis other psalms) is unimportant. My discussion of Psalm 38, in particular, takes into account the manner in which neighboring psalms shed light on Psalm 38 and so affect our reading of it. I have chosen to read the psalms in this particular, noncanonical order because this arrangement reflects the processual, non-linear nature of the experience of pain.

Psalm 69 is a fitting place to begin because it expresses and addresses at least three characteristics common to the experience of pain. One of these characteristics is the systemic nature of pain, which can seem overwhelming. Psalm 69 opens with a description of the psalmist's condition as a whole-person problem, evocatively portrayed with water metaphors to denote its overwhelming nature. That the psalm does not begin with the onset of illness or pain reflects that the feeling of being overwhelmed often comes only after dealing with the pain for some time and signals the whole-person effect of the event. A person in pain seldom appreciates the systemic effect of the pain until he or she has realized that it is not merely an odd aberration in his or her life that will soon be gone and can be forgotten. It has become a part of the pained person's life and self. Such realization can be both terribly depressing and critical to healing, to the process of reintegration.

Another basic characteristic of a person's experience of pain is the search for meaning. Why this pain? Why me?

Psalm 69 is dominated by the psalmist's concern with reasons, and this concern draws readers in to the process of interpretation. Having noted that other people add to her pain for no reason, the psalmist goes on to express concern that by reason of her suffering, others will lose faith in God. The psalmist develops this further by telling that her pain is actually on account of God—that by behaving in a "right" manner, she has elicited taunts, ridicule, and scorn. Furthermore, the psalmist appeals to God's reputation for reasons why God should come to her aid. Finally, the psalm concludes by suggesting that the psalmist suffers on account of others and this provides some reason for the psalmist's pain. By suffering as she has, the psalmist has gained the authority to encourage others and so to alleviate their pain.

A third characteristic of the experience of pain, and one that informs the other two in Psalm 69, is the role that others have in affecting the nature of the experience. It describes the social condition of the pained person and its effect on his or her experience. It does so by telling the devastating effects of rejection and scorn, expressing concern for how the psalmist's pain might adversely affect others, explicitly naming a couple of ways that others can help a person in pain (and how others might fail in that), and finally by demonstrating how a pained person's experience might help others. This relational characteristic is an underappreciated aspect of the experience of pain today, at least in the highly individualistic condition of North American society. Many of the psalms reflect the fact that one's social circumstances affect one's experience of pain, both for good and ill. Psalm 69 raises issues of the role of other persons—the Other who exacerbates pain, the Other who does (not) express sympathy and care for the pained person, and the suffering Other who finds comfort and encouragement from the psalmist's expressions and thoughts about the experience.

Psalm 38 picks up the matter of meaning, seeking reasons for the pain in another, quite common way. The author of Psalm 38 reflects one interpretation of pain as the just punishment of God for one's wrongdoing. Psalm 38 does not conclude there, however, but presses the issue by telling how the pain itself has become problematic. Consequently, the psalmist declares that God need not punish any more and actually ought to come to the psalmist's aid. The speaker of Psalm 38 is not finally content to accept the pain as punishment, but calls for an end to it and is entirely unapologetic about asking for God's help (theoretically to save the psalmist from God's own action). Although it tells of the distance and/or active malice of others as contributing to the psalmist's dire circumstances, it differs from Psalm 69 in part by not calling for vengeance. Instead, Psalm 38 describes in more detail the particular condition of the psalmist's pain, and it concentrates only on God. It does not shift its address from God.

The first two psalms, in the order that I have determined to discuss them, address the matter of meaning. This is one of the primary and most striking issues for a person in pain. In Psalm 69, the issue of interpretation is multilayered; in Psalm 38, the simple equation of pain as punishment is accepted, then challenged and complicated. Neither of these finally determines a single, hard-and-fast reason that explains the psalmist's experience of pain. Sometimes people despair of ever determining the bases and purposes for their pain, finding in the experience nothing redeeming, nothing sensible, nothing comforting. Psalm 88 in its darkness, expresses both persistent loyalty to God and frustration at the lack of response and care from God and from others. The psalmist's tone is angry and heartbroken, identifying God as the one behind her senseless suffering, which includes (and concludes with) expression of social isolation. I discuss Psalm 88 as the third of the six psalms for a couple of reasons. The sense of despair that Psalm 88 tells is seldom immediate for a person in pain, but usually follows a frustrated search for meaning, and so I follow discussion of Psalms 69 and 38 with that of Psalm 88. Furthermore, many psalms concerning pain have, somewhere in the middle, a turning-point expression, which often signals a lowest point, the nadir of the experience. Situated in the middle of the six psalms that I discuss in this book, and ending with loneliness and darkness, Psalm 88 represents the nadir of pain.

The next in my ordering, Psalm 22, begins with such profound loneliness, but it also includes a sense of abandonment by God. It follows well on the conclusion of Psalm 88, which sustains speech to God throughout. With the desperate cry of Psalm 22, "My God, my God, why have you abandoned me," dark loneliness reaches its most severe pitch. The psalmist of Psalm 22 tells not only of isolation from the community and abandonment by God but also of self-rejection, the feeling of being subhuman, cut off even from the human species. The experience of chronic pain, as it goes on and on, leaves many people truly alone. Sometimes it is accompanied by a sense of terror, even anticipation of attack on an already terribly compromised self. Regaining the self-respect that allows one to feel worthwhile as a human being, and finding a place within a greater community of people is crucial to the process of healing, whether or not it is accompanied by cure. Psalm 22 concludes with such a positive expression. Because its first part is so despairing and pained and its second part is so confident and celebratory, many scholars suppose that it was originally two psalms. Whatever the case, we have one psalm now, with two quite different parts. Psalm 22 not only follows well on Psalm 88, by picking up the tone of desperation and sense of abandonment, but it also anticipates well the reintegration of self and self-in-community that spells relief from pain.

Similar in its sense of attention to something other than the pain, Psalm 6 demonstrates a process of moving pain out from the center of the pained person's experience and thinking. I have placed Psalm 6 at this point because it does not allow us to resolve the condition of pain neatly (as concluding with Psalm 22 might do), but keeps the problem alive and present. In doing so, however, it also reflects the relief of a change of focus, or even more, of locating in the pained person's life things other than his or her pain. Consequently, reading and discussing Psalm 6 in this situation, following the discussions of Psalms 69, 38, 88, and 22, acknowledges that pain and its attendant issues are seldom finally resolved but instead may continue to be a source of distress. Nevertheless, pain's continuing presence need not preclude standing up for oneself and "talking back" to the pain.

I conclude with Psalm 102 because it concerns the finitude of a person's life by comparison with the eternal nature of God. The experience of pain is a reminder of human limits and frequently represents a kind of death. Although death is inevitable, the poet of Psalm 102 mourns the passing of his life and in so doing, even in the context of illness and pain, speaks of the value and desirability of life. Again in this psalm, the speaker tells of loneliness, community, and God's care for those who suffer. These are themes that reiterate aspects of the experience of pain as articulated in the psalms and attested by those who suffer. Its attention to the inevitability of death and to the eternalness of God makes Psalm 102 a fitting conclusion to this discussion of particular psalms in the context of an inquiry into pain, its expression and relief. However, it also is a fitting conclusion because readers will note similarities to Psalm 69, the first in my study. That is, as conclusion, it draws attention back to beginnings, demonstrating the non-linear experience of pain. It is not as though one could identify particular stages that a person goes through in suffering and seeking relief from pain; rather, questions of meaning continue to arise in different contexts: the sense of loneliness and abandonment recurs, the search for relief by telling the pain and hoping in the compassion and care of others, the acknowledgment of life's intrinsic worth and the self as an integrated person, and exhausted desperation may all appear and reappear throughout the experience. These psalms, then, demonstrate the search for wholeness of self and self in relation to others in the context of a messy management of the challenges that pain brings. I have chosen to discuss Psalms 6, 22, 38, 69, 88, and 102 in an order that reflects the dynamic and non-linear nature of the experience of pain while covering a wide range of expressions out of and through suffering. Reading these psalms is to participate, it is both to witness and to experience a being for others.

Please note: my translation of these psalms is available at the back of the book.

4

On Whose Account, This Pain and Its Relief? (Psalm 69)

"I have sunk in the mire of the deeps, and there is no place to stand; I have come in to the depths of the water and rushing streams dash over me."

Chronic pain, by definition, does not have a clear beginning. Or, more accurately, its beginning can be identified, if at all, only after great suffering. Defined by duration, such pain is notable only after one has wrestled with it and with its effects on the innumerable aspects of a single life. The recognition that pain is not going away any time soon is a turning-point in the experience. Often accompanied by feelings of exhaustion, anger, and despair, this recognition is a kind of beginning as one acknowledges the manner in which pain affects all aspects of the self, and so realizes that one must make sense of it in the context of the totality of one's life if one is to be whole. I begin the discussion of psalms with Psalm 69 in part because it reflects these characteristics. It does not begin with a description of injury or the onset of suffering, and only late in the psalm cites pain explicitly (verse 29). Rather, it begins with an exclamation that marks a turning-point in the experience, and it demonstrates that a part of the nature of this turning-point is the struggle to make sense of the pain.

We as readers not only witness the process but also experience for ourselves the dynamic, trial-and-error nature of interpretation in the context of a multifaceted life. In Psalm 69, the cry of one who has suffered long and hard and the preoccupation with reasons for such pain are interconnected. Furthermore, the psalm shows that the systemic nature of pain and the struggle to make sense of it are informed, for good and ill, by the sufferer's relationships — by his or her social circumstances.

Psalm 69 takes us on an excavation of the ruins of pain. Its strata and the range of interpretations that grow out of inquiring after their meanings are reflected in the variety of roles that other people play. All references to reason and meaning in Psalm 69 are associated with particular relationships to others. This is first expressed by identification of wrongful accusers and attackers (reason or cause for the most problematic aspect of pain), then in concern for their effect on attitudes of the psalmist's community — that those who identify with the psalmist would also experience shame and lose faith (reason for God to save the psalmist from pain). Then, meanings become associated with description of the failure of others to relieve the psalmist's pain (reason for worsening pain), followed by a desire for the enemies' undoing in vengeance against those who caused the psalmist pain (reason for others' pain). Finally, the psalmist is concerned to witness to others about God's saving action and participate in a community of praise (reason or purpose for both pain and its relief).

A New Beginning and the Search for Reasons

"Save me, O God, for the waters have come in to my very self. I am mired in the mud of the deeps, and there is nowhere to stand." Drowning with the exhaustion of living in pain, the sufferer's condition surpasses a purely "physical" problem, one that might be addressed and cured. The psalmist cries out, "the waters have broached my very self," announcing that the terrifying sensation affects her whole being—her *nephesh*, in Hebrew, a word that can be translated as "soul, self, person." By telling the overwhelming, disintegrating effects of her suffering, the poet of Psalm 69 acknowledges that pain is a whole-self event and demands a whole-self address. We know nothing of the psalmist's pain before this exclamation of distress, and we learn few of the details that would describe the particularity of her suffering. Instead, the psalm starts with recognition that the pain is not going away. The poet cries out that she "can no more." Exhaustion, frustration, and despair permeate Psalm 69's opening lines. They explicitly and evocatively describe the systemic nature of the experience and tell that any help must take into account the whole person suffering. Speaking from the psalmist's lowest point, she sees that the pain is not going away and that its effects have already been greatly destructive, like chaotic waters threatening her very being and smothering her vitality. Security and stability elude, as the one in pain finds no help in response to her cries and faces the danger of utter dissolution. The psalmist concludes this initial complaint by saying, "my throat is parched, my eyes are done-in, waiting for my God"—short lines that belie the kind of introversion that accompanies profound exhaustion and despair of coming help.

The beginning of the psalm tells the beginning of a new reckoning with pain. From this terrible, low place, the psalmist presses for reasons, for an interpretation of her condition in the whole of her life. "Before illness, the patient identifies with her body, with her community, and with the ultimate. [. . .] When the medical staff has finished its work and snatched the patient from the jaws of biological death, the agony has just begun. [. . .] She may need to invent, discover, and receive, minute by minute, the person moving through a mined and stricken field."[1] Only by including the experience of chronic pain in the sufferer's self-story can he or she hope to craft an honest, albeit dynamic, understanding of his or her life. And only by integrating the pain into such an understanding can the sufferer reintegrate the fractured pieces of his or her self. With sustained pain, "restitution narratives" fall apart.[2] That is, dismissing illness and/or pain as a temporary interruption, nothing more than an aberration in an otherwise whole and sensible life, becomes less and less possible as pain continues to disrupt and disable. The pain has become a(n insensible) part of that life.

Therefore, a critical part of the process of reintegrating the self is fashioning an understanding of that particular life that accounts for and makes sense of the continuing presence of pain. It is no surprise, then, that the author of Psalm 69 is concerned with reasons to such a degree and in such variety as to seem preoccupied, or even obsessed with finding and defining them—reasons for the pain, her suffering as reason for others to lose faith, reasons for God to address the psalmist's suffering, and her suffering as reason for others to have hope. Simply listing these reasons shows the wide-ranging nature of the psalmist's struggle for and with meaning and hints at its inseparability from matters of relationship with others and with God. Attending to this struggle, as we do by reading and discussing the psalm, is to witness an important part of the reintegration that characterizes healing.

Psalm 69 not only makes its readers witnesses, however, but it also makes of us participants in the process of meaning-making. It makes us complicit in the process, inviting us to investigate and conjecture. The conclusions we draw early in our reading are tempered, altered, and challenged by subsequent lines. Wittingly or not, we discover that there are layers to the psalmist's pain. As these layers become evident, we find that our interpretation must be a process, accommodating new information into the search for reasons and meaning. Indeed, the psalmist's story, as it is revealed in these lines, develops piece by piece; and we, as readers, experience a "trying on" of interpretations, experimenting with reasons for the psalmist's pain and reasons for its relief.[3]

Such experimenting with reasons and meaning demonstrates not only the necessity of trying but also of acknowledging that interpretations are imperfect, that they require constant reassessment, tweaking, and reshaping. Recognizing the imperfect, dynamic nature of meaning-making out of pain allows us to question and challenge reasoning that finally seems not to promote the reintegration necessary to relief or healing. Nevertheless, such experimentation is the exception more often than the rule; most of us want to determine one, final reason for pain. Taking inventory of the most common interpretations, Schmidt notes that answers frequently revolve around either how closely God should be identified with the suffering or simply how or who God is. He writes of the popular, yet ultimately untenable and even destructive "cold comforts" that people frequently propose as though finally to answer the problem of pain. They include ideas such as "we suffer because we sin," "suffering is God's will," "God uses suffering to teach us," "we suffer because we don't pray or don't have faith in God," and "God doesn't will us to suffer but allows us to suffer."[4]

Psalm 69 does not permit readers to settle easily into such answers and actually undermines each of them. It draws readers into the experience of "trying on" interpretations, "trying on" reasons for the pain, and "trying on" reasons for its relief as descriptions of the psalmist's complaints and description of her condition lead readers into constantly changing interpretations. Psalm 69 reveals layers of pain that require layers of meaning-making. Without necessarily setting out to do so, readers modify and adjust reasons for the psalmist's pain and reasons for its relief as they integrate new information, line by line, into a developing sense of the psalmist's experience.

Excavating the Layers of Pain

The opening lines, with their expression of great torment and despair, make readers wonder why the psalmist suffers so. Following the psalmist's initial complaint of exhaustion and despair, she draws God's (and the reader's) attention to the deceit and malice of others. "Many more than the hairs on my head are those who hate me for no reason. Vast are those who would annihilate me, my deceitful enemies." Given this complaint, immediately following the psalmist's exclamation of suffering, we conjecture that she suffers because of these other people who threaten and wrongly accuse her of criminal activity. Indeed, the literary position of this complaint leads to an interpretation that these other people may be the reason for the psalmist's pain ironically *because there is no reason* for their hatred and ill-wishes. The rhetorical question that follows, "Should I give back what I have not taken?" hints that their antagonism is due to a belief that the psalmist has robbed something from them. That she is innocent leads readers to conclude that there is no (good) reason for the psalmist to suffer and that her pain is directly due to the attack of others.

In the movie, *Philadelphia*, Tom Hanks plays Andrew Beckett, a promising, young, "razor-sharp," lawyer, rising in the ranks of a prestigious law firm. Darling of the firm's partners, we witness his promotion and hear the praise and confidence his work has evoked among the firm's leaders. Soon after facial lesions make Beckett's AIDS visible, important work that he had done is inexplicably misplaced, and he is dismissed from the practice. The partners who had been so solicitous of Beckett become his attackers. On trumped up charges, they fire him. Of course the reasons that they give have nothing to do with his illness; instead they claim that he has been irresponsible and done poor work. At first, Beckett is overwhelmed and bewildered by their decision. It does not make sense. There are layers to this pain-the pain of the illness itself and the pain that others inflict on account of the illness. While the first layer of pain may have a meaningful reason (the assault of viruses on a body without defense), the other's reason is no reason.

Just as there are layers to Beckett's pain, so we discover that there are layers to the psalmist's pain, with consequent layers to its reasons and meaning that are not immediately evident. Indeed, only after listening to the whole story can we appreciate them. At first, the psalmist's distress seems to have a definable, though unjustified, cause —the attack of others who make erroneous accusations of criminal activity and who then presume to punish to such a degree that the psalmist fears annihilation at their hands. That is there is no reason for the accusation and attack of these others complicates the psalmist's pain.

However, the next line, "O God, you know my folly, and my wrongdoing is not concealed from you," demands that readers accommodate the fact that the psalmist is not innocent. Although innocent of the charges that others bring against her, she acknowledges that she is guilty of other (unidentified) things. Acceding another layer to the psalmist's pain, we may abandon our earlier supposition that it is due to the malice of other people and conclude that she suffers primarily the pain of deserved punishment for some unnamed crime. However, this interpretation also demands immediate reassessment, for the psalmist appeals to God for help out of an honest recognition that she is not blameless. In so doing, the psalmist calls into question the idea that her pain is simply punishment and so should be accepted. Indeed, the psalm challenges not only the notion that suffering is payment for sin but also that suffering is God's will. The psalmist claims that she suffers *despite* her wrongdoing and fiercely requests (and expects) help, thereby proposing that God does not desire such suffering for the psalmist and should not allow it. That the psalmist claims that others might suffer on account of her suffering underscores the conclusion that her pain is finally unjustified. "Do not let those who hope in you be shamed on account of me [. . .] Do not let those who seek you be humiliated because of me," the psalmist says.

This suggests yet another layer of the psalmist's pain, a layer developed in the next verses where we learn that the psalmist suffers destructive humiliation because of her integrity vis-à-vis God. "On account of you I have put up with scorn," the psalmist cries. But it is an integrity that includes honest recognition of previous failings. The psalmist does not claim to be blameless, only that this particular suffering has nothing to do with accountability to God. Indeed, the *problematic* pain at issue in the psalmist's complaint is the pain that other people have caused her. Sorry about some unnamed, earlier "folly" and "wrongdoing," the psalmist explains that she wept, fasted, and wore sackcloth, all demonstrations of repentance. But the psalmist protests that because of these outward signs of right action, others made of her a morality lesson, gossiped, and made jokes about her.

As the psalmist uncovers layers of her pain, our interpretations become more nuanced, allowing that the pain that threatens to destroy the psalmist's very self, the pain that drives her to beg for help is not the pain of just punishment from God. On the contrary, it is the pain of social rejection in the context of a suffering out of integrity. Citing a number of studies done by psychiatric researchers, the medical anthropologists who wrote *Pain as Human Experience: An Anthropological Perspective* observe, "Depression and anxiety, serious family tensions, conflicted work relationships—all conduce to the onset or exacerbation of chronic pain conditions and, in turn, may be worsened by chronic pain. Physical pain complaints therefore express painful relations and experiences."[5] While there is some general condition of pain, as noted in the psalmist's brief exclamation in verse 29, "I am afflicted and in pain," it is the pain suffered at the hands or mouths of others that dis-integrates the psalmist. The problematic pain is not, then, purely physical, but is associated with her social situation and has psychological and spiritual implications.

Having suffered the humiliation and career-destruction of being fired from the most prestigious law firm in Philadelphia, Andrew Beckett determines to sue the practice for unjustly dismissing him. Initially rejected by Denzel Washington's character, attorney Joe Miller, Beckett sets out to prepare the case himself. When he and Miller meet again, it is in the library where both are working. Wrestling to overcome his repulsion of Beckett, Miller listens as Beckett describes the bases on which they will win the case. The Federal Vocational Rehabilition Act of 1973, issued in defense of disabled persons, provides precedence. Beckett notes that its wording includes AIDS victims "because prejudice surrounding AIDS exacts a social death which precedes the actual physical one."

The failure of others to sympathize, comfort, and care for the patient, or worse yet their propensity to blame them for his or her condition heaps insult on the injury and can exacerbate the physical experience of pain. The article "Does Rejection Hurt? An fMRI Study of Social Exclusion," published in the journal *Science*, explains that recent neuroimaging studies actually demonstrate that social separation or rejection has the same physiological effects as physical pain does.[6] Note how speech complicates and exacerbates the psalmist's pain. The speech of others scorning, condemning, and gossiping is more hurtful to the psalmist than any "sticks and stones."

It is this kind of torment that the psalmist fears for others who are like her. "Do not let those who hope in you (God) be shamed on account of me [. . .] Do not let those who seek you be humiliated because of me." Conditions that are difficult to diagnose and become associated with particular stereotypes threaten to dehumanize sufferers of the stereotyped group. Because temporomandibular joint (TMJ) problems elicit pains varying in site, intensity, and duration, TMJ is difficult to diagnose and to treat. Sufferers frequently endure years of differing diagnoses and treatments that often exacerbate their pain and even call into question their sanity. The psalmist fears that her pain will become reason for the embarrassment and humiliation that others might suffer because of a likeness to her. The psalmist is concerned that if one such as she suffers the reproach and attacks of others because of her loyalty to God and refusal to give up on defining principles in her life, then others who look to her as a model may also grow demoralized and/or suffer similarly. Mary

Bartlett, who links her experiences of years in pain to TMJ explains, "I just hope my history gets out there to help someone else. No one should have to live in this turmoil and be told there is nothing wrong with them."[7] Similarly, Gail Johnston says, "It's so frustrating to be legitimately ill and have people treating you as though [. . .] you're just another crazy female."[8]

The high-profile lawsuit that Beckett brings against his former employers elicits great public demonstrations against homosexuality and a parade of "cold comfort" interpretations of AIDS. Although Beckett and Miller win the case, it is a long and exhausting process for Beckett whose condition worsens throughout the course of the trial. We see how Beckett's experience with AIDS has not only wide-ranging physical implications, but also takes a terrific emotional and social toll. This social toll, the exacerbation of pain because of others, includes not only social rejection, scorn, and ridicule but also concern for those who identify with him. "Tongues wag" and all sorts of rumors about the sufferer's behavior circulate. The person pained by AIDS becomes a lesson for others and the subject of all sorts of unsavory stories, jokes, and assumptions. Under vicious attack from those who interpret the condition as the result of sinful behavior, Beckett also expresses concern for how such abuse might affect his partner, others in the gay community, and his supportive family.

A variety of relationships inform the layers of the psalmist's pain and are bound up together in it. Others who add to the psalmist's pain do so in direct relation to her innocence; and the psalmist expresses concern that others who identify with the psalmist will likewise suffer. Furthermore, these factors—the psalmist's innocence and the roles of others—not only determine the shape of the psalmist's pain but also are bound up in reasons the psalmist proposes that God should help her: lest enemies think that they are right, and lest those who look to the psalmist as a model lose hope or faith and suffer the scorn and ridicule that so torments the psalmist.

Development of Interpretations, Turning Attention toward Others

These relationships inform the second half of the psalm, too, where the psalmist develops their implications. That the psalmist returns to the imagery of overwhelming waters immediately after her complaint about mistreatment by others attests to the role of these others as critical to the psalmist's condition. Furthermore, in this second plea for help from entrapping mud and threatening waters the psalmist adds, "let me be rescued from those who hate me." By this halfway point in the psalm, we have considered layers of the psalmist's pain and determined that we must both reckon with the role of others as definitive contributors to the psalmist's pain and take into account the psalmist's concern for others who suffer.

Although we find in Psalm 69 both bases that Schmidt identified for cold comfort interpretations — God's role in the suffering and characteristics of God — they are subsumed by concern with relationships. That is, concerning God's role, the psalmist does say "on account of you (God), I suffer," yet God's role in informing the psalmist's experience of her pain is secondary to the roles of other people. Similarly, although the psalmist appeals to the character of God as reason for help, ("Because of your abundant kindness [. . .] according to your abundant compassion,"), she does so in direct relation to the effect that such help would have on others, both those who torment her, that they would not be vindicated, and those who look to the psalmist as a model, that they would not be shamed. Psalm 69 requires that we temper interpretations of the psalmist's pain that are based on ideas about the degree of God's role in suffering and characteristics of God with the powerful influence that other people have. Indeed, as the psalm continues, it becomes clear that the psalmist's relationships inform her experience of pain more than anything else does.

The most problematic aspect of the psalmist's pain seems to be the scorn and ridicule of those who claim that the psalmist is guilty of something and who make fun of her and of her distress. Not only does the psalm demonstrate that blamelessness is not a required condition to appeal for help, but it also criticizes those who would argue that pain is the just result of some sin or other, and thereby add to the suffering.[9] The psalm challenges the idea that pain is punishment for some sin; instead, it lays primary responsibility for the psalmist's suffering at the feet, hands, and mouths of other people. This psalm not only refutes an interpretation that pain is God's means of instruction or punishment but it also proposes that human pain is the purview of other people—they sometimes exacerbate and always should seek to relieve it.

One way that people have made sense of the end of the book of Job, with God's seemingly irrelevant response to Job's complaint, is by suggesting that God makes the problem of Job's suffering the responsibility of other people. Rather than sit around trying to figure out what Job did wrong, his companions ought to have been trying to alleviate his suffering. Indeed, God's accusation of Job's friends at the end of the book is that they did not speak about God correctly, as Job did. While Job persisted in his integrity, challenging and even criticizing God, his friends looked on in horror at what they felt to be gross and dangerous irreverence. Nevertheless, it is Job that God finds to be in the right, and only Job's appeal on his friend's behalf can save them from God's consequent punishment of them. The two occasions of "you know" in Psalm 69 identify basic layers of the psalmist's pain and underscore the sense that, despite relation with God perhaps in the context of pain, her relationship with malicious others is the source of problematic pain. The "you know" of verse 5, concerning the psalmist's wrongdoing, becomes the "you know" of verse 19 concerning the pain suffered by social rejection.

It is no wonder that a person in such a condition might feel angry and bitter toward those who not only refuse to help but who also attempt to justify the person's pain, perhaps even humiliating him or her because of it. It is no wonder that such a person would wish on his or her tormenters the same experience of pain and isolation. The psalmist presumes that theirs is the crime of humiliating and wrongly judging another out of a presumption to see and speak as God. Consequently, disturbing though these exclamations of a desire for vengeance are, it is understandable that the psalmist would ask that God punish these others who do her such harm.

Is That Really in the Bible?!

These expressions of desire for vengeance, sometimes violent and even cruel, deserve special mention here not least because they are quite common in psalms concerning pain, although we rarely take note of them. There is a tendency in biblical scholarship as well as personal devotion to overlook, ignore, or dismiss these expressions.[10] That we have an aversion to them is probably a good sign of hesitation to do violence to others. However, David Mamet notes, "The Torah acknowledges that unpleasant and destructive feelings cannot be wished away, they must be examined and dealt with."[11] Indeed, there are several matters that commend these disturbing expressions for further attention.

One is the necessity for justice. A world in which crimes and abuses are committed with impunity is chaotic at best, bedeviled at worst. Those of us lucky enough to have been spared victimization at the hands of others are inclined to dismiss the violent acts of others if the perpetrators express even a hint of remorse. But one wonders if it is anyone's place, who was not the victim, to forgive. Such forgiveness by others than the one hurt can have a deleterious effect on the actual victim. The Korean word *han* describes just such a condition. *Han* is the pain of the victim. It cannot be assuaged by others' forgiveness of the one who did harm and can actually be exacerbated by such forgiveness. In his book *The Wounded Heart of God*, Andrew Sung Park explains that without addressing *han*, a victim of violence may well go on to commit the same assault against someone else.[12] Punishment of criminal activity and vengeance against an abuser may be necessary not only to prevent the same from happening again but also to attempt to redress the wrong in such a way that the victim gains some relief. Further, without such relief, the victim may go on, in bitterness, disillusionment, and anger (toward self and others) to become perpetrator of more criminal activity. Mercy has its place, but so too does justice.[13]

This brings me to my second point about these difficult texts: their presence requires our engagement with them, even (perhaps especially) if we determine to reject their sentiments. In this way, they may be considered a kind of schoolroom for moral and ethical reasoning and debate. By stirring in us feelings of repulsion to and rejection of them, we practice human freedom to exercise intelligence and choice, to weigh our propensity to do another harm against decisions to halt cyclical violence. Such texts stimulate debate and resistance, promoting skills of reasoning and argument that preclude taking damaging action against another. Perhaps a value of such texts is the manner in which they press us to say, "No. That is inappropriate, cruel, unacceptable. I will not do such a thing." Indeed, note that the psalmist does not take action against hurtful others.

Another reason that such texts commend themselves to us for consideration is that they allow a cathartic expression of very real reactionary wishes for vengeance, born of anger, disappointment, rejection, hurt.[14] Sometimes it is necessary to tell such feelings, to "let them out," in order to be rid of them. That is, by giving voice to such disturbing, even hateful, thoughts, one may find relief from them. It is significant that they are not addressed to the hurtful party but are directed to God. Addressing such thoughts only to God means that they "stop there," rather than infecting the thinking and behavior of others toward the hated person or group. Furthermore, they *can* stop there because they are said, not done. The matter of solving the issue becomes God's problem. Notice that the speaker in such psalmic texts does not take matters into his or her own hands; instead, it becomes the business of God to determine how to exact vengeance, if at all.

Furthermore, in addition to providing legitimacy and an outlet for such feelings, actually hearing oneself say them can abort the desire to act on them. The effect can be humblingly surprising. Sometimes, expressing wishes for violence on another person creates a backlash effect. One hears the horror of it and any desire to act on the wishes vanishes. A man in the midst of an ugly divorce exclaimed to me that he wished that the airplane his ex-wife was on would fall out of the sky. No sooner had the words left his mouth than his eyes widened in horror, and he whispered, "What a terrible thing to say. I don't wish anything of the sort." Sometimes saying such things out loud is all that's needed to be rid of the feeling.

Taking God out of the Reasoning — Relief in Being for Others

In the center of the psalm, which returns to the chaotic water imagery that introduced the psalmist's plight, the psalmist cries again for help out of the mess and again speaks of the whole - person nature of the psalmist's dire condition: "come close to my soul/self; rescue it." Again, the Hebrew term *nephesh* is the object of concern. That this word also connotes "passion, desire, emotion" further testifies to the systemic effect of the psalmist's pain. Indeed, characteristics of a vital self that demonstrate full engagement in the world include passion, desire, and emotion. Conversely, a person suffering great and lasting pain frequently experiences a profound depression that flattens passion and desire. Not all desire is productive, but some is necessary for life itself. Nevertheless, suffering leads one to wonder: given this constant pain, this unremitting illness, what is the point. A kind of resignation, not to the reality of continuing pain and/or illness, but to the loss of what gave one a sense of purpose and worth, can make fulfilling the most mundane needs seem wasteful: why buy groceries, wear sunscreen, take a shower. Cancer sufferer, Anatole Broyard, calls this "falling out of love with yourself," and advises thinking of great pain and constant illness as permission to do what you have enjoyed and/or wanted to do.[15]

The challenge for a person facing such feelings is to resist the flood waters of pain that threaten to sweep away the productive desire that enables life. This productive, life-affirming desire manifests itself not simply in promot-

ing behavior that enables an individual life, but also in
being for others, in extending the love of self to love for
others, all who share the human experience of pain.[16]
Furthermore, this manner of being out of one's suffering
for others who suffer can bring with it its own relief. As
the psalm continues, we find that the psalmist's exclamation and process of searching for and describing meaning
exemplifies being for others both in telling pain *as* pain
and in developing a narrative that accounts for pain's part
in a person's whole self. We find that in being for others
the psalmist's tone changes from complaint to satisfaction
and confidence.

Gail Johnston explains that the suffering she has
endured on account of TMJ—physical, psychological,
and emotional—has reoriented her life from a desire to
stand out as a brilliant professor and academic leader to a
desire simply to be for others, both those who are in pain
and those who are not. She explains, "I can't help but feel
like [. . .] not that there's a purpose to my pain, but that I
haven't let it triumph. I've made it into something else.
I've made it into a way to make connections to people."[17]
Painting and drawing out of her pain, Gail makes these
connections to others, encouraging those who are in pain
and instructing others about pain; and she explains that
this purposeful process brings satisfaction and relief.
"[Pain] is like a shadow that throws the other parts of my
life into brighter contrast [. . .] [B]ecause I have this darkness hovering all around the edges [. . .] the world has
become a more precious and beautiful place—because I
really see it."[18]

Although the psalm draws readers into the kind of reasoning that lies behind the cold comforts that Schmidt
describes, it tells neither how responsible God is for the
psalmist's pain nor what God is like. "When, at long last,

the reality of the pain and loss that accompanies suffering is admitted — when we are candid — then faith continues to be possible only if those who suffer are given a different means of thinking about God."[19] In his groundbreaking book, *Otherwise than Being or Beyond Essence*, twentieth-century French philosopher Emmanuel Levinas describes his presumption that there is something basic to being human that assumes responsibility for the other, an other person who is appreciated as distinct, yet with whom one is in relationship and for whose well-being one assumes responsibility. He notes that a theology reflective of the Hebrew Bible must account for this relational nature of human beings and observes the priority of relationship to others in any Jewish theology. In contrast with what he identifies as a characteristically Christian emphasis on an individual's direct encounter with God, he writes, "As Jews, we are always a threesome: I and you and the Third who is in our midst. And only as a Third does He reveal Himself."[20] This thinking is inseparable from thinking about others. Despite sustained attention to the relationship between the psalmist and God and how that relationship informs the psalmist's condition, the psalm concludes by focusing on the psalmist's "being-for" relationship to others, and its change of speech actually demonstrates relationship: the final part of the psalm is addressed to other people.

Although the psalmist has led us to "try on" interpretations that contribute to the kind of meaning-making that relies on ideas of God's role in the suffering and/or the character of God, the psalm finally moves away from the why questions to concentrate on other people, those who exacerbate and those who are in or are at risk of pain. The last statement of pain that the psalmist makes stands between her vitriolic request that God punish those who have made her pain what it is and her address to others within her community. It is simple and brief: "I am afflicted and in pain." There is no reasoning, and no invitation for further interpretation from readers. The psalmist does not dispute any of the reasons that we have tried on in the course of reading the psalm, but neither are we allowed to conclude that there is one answer. Instead of continuing to wrestle with the pain and attempts to find meaning for it in the context of address to God, attention turns to other people, and the tone brightens. Out of the author's pain she addresses others who suffer as well as the whole universe, and in the process both demonstrates relationship to God in enjoyment of and delight with the world and encourages those in pain to seek help and have confidence that they are not alone, ignored, or dismissed in their pain.

Although previous verses concerned other people, they were addressed to God. Despite attention to the enemies that so dominated the first part of the psalm, the last section is addressed to others of the psalmist's community. By contrast to the psalm's earlier tone of complaint and desire for vengeance, this last part is dominated by a tone of thanksgiving and hopefulness. The psalm changes from complaint to God to praise of God, hope, and encouragement for others. At the end, the psalmist reaches out to others in pain and suffering, encouraging them and expressing confidence in their relief. The psalmist's suffering justifies her words to them and enables her to establish a relationship that supports and strengthens others who suffer. In so doing, the psalmist's tone reflects a new vitality and hope. A Buddhist meditation on suffering, expressed by Tenzin Gyatso, the fourteenth and present Dalai Lama, reflects the idea that one's suffering and how one might grow in it should not be purely personal. He proposes, instead, adopting an attitude of engagement with others who are also in pain and suggests the prayer, "May the suffering I am undergoing serve to counter the sufferings experienced by other sentient beings."[21]

Despite the historical and geographical specificity of the final lines of the psalm—possibly looking forward to a time when the war-ravaged and depopulated Judah, especially Jerusalem, will bustle with life and prosperity again—they tell something timeless, too. Attention to and concern for others, when one faces pain and suffering, reveals an orientation to the future. Levinas explains that in one's awareness of the mystery, which is the presence of death in suffering, one is able to find in the other a future. "The other is the future. The very relationship with the other is the relationship with the future."[22] Although pain can foster both self-centeredness and a reckoning with the inevitability of one's death, it simultaneously allows the sufferer to see his or her self in relationship with those who are absolutely other.[23] Psalm 69 demonstrates that responsibility in relationship goes both ways. It includes that of the sufferer to others as well as the responsibility of others to the sufferer.

The psalm does not answer the questions: why suffering? and why its relief? Neither, however, does it discount such inquiry. "Closure is a concept foreign to Jewish tradition," David Mamet notes in his reflections with Lawrence Kushner on the beginning of Genesis. "It is an overwhelmingly [. . .] arrogant idea—that one [. . .] can 'complete' a disturbing experience [. . .] The struggle to deal with an unjust, confusing, incomprehensible world does not impede our life; it is our life."[24] No systematic theology emerges from our investigation of reasons for the psalmist's pain described in Psalm 69. Rather, the psalmist's focus becomes relationships. It is only out of that condition that a "theology of candor" can develop, a theology that takes into account the reality of pain and suffering and allows for the possibility that God is first and foremost about relationships.[25]

The psalmist seems to suggest that God's interest in relationship is more definitive than abstractions of power or goodness. Or more precisely, "the goodness of God is defined in terms of God's passion for relationship and willingness to endure the ragged edges of a world in which [. . .] the variables introduced by autonomy shape the world in which God seeks us."[26] A theology of candor, honestly noting the existence and effects of pain and suffering, develops in reaction to the failure of cold comfort reasoning and reflects a powerful emphasis on relationships, especially in the context of such pain and suffering. In reading Psalm 69, we experience the necessary process of meaning-making in the face of great pain. However, rather than propose a simple solution to the problem, the psalmist takes us on an excavation—plumbing the layers of pain and trying on different interpretations. Finally, without discounting the process that preceded, the psalmist concludes with something quite other—concern for other people and the critical role that relationships play in the experience of pain.

5

From Justified Pain
to Self-Justification (Psalm 38)

✑

"O Lord, all my longing is before you, and my sighing is not hidden from you."

Twisted and bent, disconsolate, and on the verge of utterly breaking down, the author of Psalm 38 cries out. Yet despite this miserable condition, appealing for relief is not the cry's primary expression; rather, telling the real conditions of his pain dominates the psalm. In doing so, the psalmist both justifies pain and reckons with mercy. That is, the psalmist interprets the genesis and purpose of his pain as corrective punishment for wrongdoing, but tells the horrible effects of it in a manner that finally undercuts the appropriateness of such punishment. By the psalm's end, the psalmist presents a self-image that justifies mercy. Recognizing that great and lasting pain can be ultimately useless and destructive promotes a sense of self that is greater than wrongdoing and deserved punishment. This recognition of pain-turned-problematic and the intrinsic value of the sufferer enables the psalmist confidently to request that God desist from punishing and save from suffering. In the process of telling the details of his suffering, the psalmist brings together competing ideas about just punishment and radical mercy, creating a tension out of which he determines that God should act on his behalf.

Walter Brueggemann observes that without challenging the "common theology" of strict justice and the legitimated structures built on such principles, it is impossible to value "the pained and the pain-bearers." In Psalm 38 we witness first a person's recognition of his pain as just punishment for wrongdoing and then the challenge to such a "relentlessly contractual theology."[1] Because the psalmist's pain is so great that it is ultimately destructive, he challenges the facile interpretation of pain as justified punishment. Detailed description of the psalmist's systemic pain and social trauma suggests that the punishing pain has become useless, or worse, destructive. Arguing against a simple, tit-for-tat theology for the occasional exercise of divine mercy, the psalmist claims to be more than his wrongdoing and pain, and pleads for demonstration of a God who is more than justice.

Attempts to understand pain by interpreting it as divine punishment for wrongdoing seem to be as old as pain itself. A Mesopotamian poem dating to 4,000 or 3,000 B.C.E. imagines the headache poetically roaming the desert to afflict the impious person, "blowing like the wind, flashing like lightning, it is loosed above and below. It cutteth off like a reed him who feareth not his god." Also from Mesopotamia, we find this poem describing activity undertaken symbolically to rid the sufferer of his or her pain:

> As this garlic is peeled off and thrown into the fire [. . .]
> So may [. . .] the sickness of my suffering, wrong-
>   doing, crime, misdeed, sin,
> The sickness which is in my body, flesh, and sinews
> Be peeled off like this garlic,
> May Girra burn it with fire this day.[2]

The ancient Greeks also promoted such interpretation in their religious stories and legends. Consider Prometheus, caught for stealing fire from the gods and condemned to have his liver eaten out by ravens every night; or Pandora whose disobedience released all of the ills that trouble human beings. In Book 1 of Homer's *Odyssey*, Zeus echoes this interpretation and subtly challenges it with a secular twist: "My word, how mortals take the gods to task! All their afflictions come from us, we hear. And what of their own failings? Greed and folly double the suffering in the lot of man."

That we also find in the Bible ideas of pain as the result of sin should come as no surprise. Ancient storytellers of Genesis narrate the disobedience of the first people and its resulting introduction of suffering and pain. This basic perspective recurs throughout the Hebrew Bible, earning the Old Testament the mistakenly narrow identity as the book(s) about a wrathful and punishing God dealing with a persistently sinful people. Such narrow theological interpretation is presumed in the New Testament, too. Basic to Christianity is the message that people are inherently sinful and their wrongdoing demands accounting or payment in pain. Reflecting its Hebrew inheritance (in the prophet Isaiah's suffering servant), Christians believe that one who is innocent may suffer vicariously the pain due others in order that these others may be set right with God. Understanding Jesus to be the means of such salvation leads many Christians consequently to prioritize Jesus' suffering above other aspects of his life and teachings. The popularity of Mel Gibson's movie, "The Passion of the Christ," which tells little else about Jesus than Gibson's interpretation of great and gruesome suffering and death, attests to the continuing power of such thinking. Interpretations of pain and suffering as punishments from God for a person or community's wrongdoing have persisted throughout history. Augustine, who was a highly influential Christian, not least because of his self-identity as a great sinner wrote, "pain in the flesh is only a discomfort of the soul arising from the flesh, and a kind of shrinking from its suffering."[3] Expressing a similar theology, the great seventeenth-century philosopher Blaise Pascal, prayed, "Move my heart so to repent my faults, since, without this internal sorrow, the external ills with which thou affectest my body will be to me a new occasion of sin. Make me truly to know that the ills of the body are nothing else than punishment and the symbol combined of the ills of the soul."[4]

A modern ambivalence about pain (does it serve some necessary purpose or should we hope and strive to eradicate it altogether?) is the subject of a lecture given in 1999 at the University of Florida College of Medicine by anesthesiologist Donald Caton.[5] Tracing ideas of pain in antiquity and into the nineteenth century (before the advent of pain-killing medications), Caton observes that pain was perceived in the western world as the result of sin, a natural state of being for all people.[6] After the introduction of medications that dulled pain and/or rendered the sufferer unconscious for the duration of an otherwise painful medical procedure, Caton notes that there was great optimism about the possibility of ridding human experience of pain completely. Pain itself came to be considered evil, and the moral language of "rights" crept into discourse about suffering with the sense that every one has a right to live without pain. Nevertheless, ideas about pain as somehow necessary, especially concerning corrective punishment, persist; and today we continue to wrestle with these opposing perspectives.

In reading Psalm 38, we find an explanation of pain as both justified punishment for breaking contract with God and reason for relief, in protest against such justification. More precisely, we witness a person's initial understanding of pain as divine punishment for his wrongdoing give way to justification for relief, a justification that does not necessitate innocence. Psalm 38 is framed by requests to God that mark the movement of this psalm from justified pain to self-justification. The first request, "do not rebuke me in your anger, nor chasten me in your rage" introduces the psalmist's interpretation of his pain as justified punishment, an interpretation confirmed by the psalmist's explicit declaration of his guilt. The only other request that the psalmist makes to God concludes the psalm with an eager plea for relief, "Do not leave me, [. . .] Do not be far from me. Hurry to my aid, my Lord, my salvation." Such a poignant expression of desire for God's proximity and help is impossible without a sense of justification in asking. That is, without a sense of self that is worthy of relief, no such request could be forthcoming. That the author concludes with attention to self (note the number of occurrences of "me" and "my") in contrast to its beginning attention to God (note the number of occurrences of "your"), further underscores the psalmist's shift from interpreting pain as deserved punishment to finding pain too problematic in its dehumanizing effects.

The requests that frame the psalm introduce the psalmist's search for the meaning of his pain in previous acts of guilt or wrongdoing and conclude with confirmation of the psalmist's movement away from such justification of pain to a simple desire for relief. Two intervening exclamations to God mark the shift, "O Lord, all my longing is before you, [. . .]" (verse 9) and "For you, YHWH, I wait; you, you will answer, my Lord, my God" (verse 15). These hope-filled exclamations are embedded in descriptions of the nature and extent of the psalmist's suffering and hint at the psalm's move away from justification of the pain toward justification in asking for relief simply because the pain is so bad. The longing for God's presence and help that permeate the psalmist's final request confirm the sense that the pain is too great and far-reaching to justify as appropriate punishment. The pain is instead destructive to the psalmist's person, and this destruction justifies his cry for help to a God whom the psalmist presumes would not will such pain.

Psalm 38's greater literary context underscores its movement from justified pain to self-justification, and it demonstrates ambivalence about the value of painful punishment in the first place. Psalm 38 reflects not only this ambivalence but also change, the development to new ways of thinking about the pain that highlight the person suffering and not simply the pain as justified punishment. In the process, we witness how initial thinking about the meaning of pain is transformed and finally undercut by a general concern for the sufferer's greater life and welfare. Interpreting one's pain initially as the just punishment for previous wrongdoing may seem appropriate and actually bring a sense of comfort with its justification. However, pain that is destructive of the self as a person and in relation to others calls into question not only any such purpose and value for pain but also any method of interpretation that is reductive of a person and of God. The author of Psalm 38 candidly demonstrates a three-fold process from initial interpretation of his pain as justified punishment, to awareness and exclamation of the ultimately destructive nature of the pain, finally to determining that as a whole person he is justified in asking that God act, support, and save him.

Even Deserved Pain Can Be Too Much

Psalm 38 begins with several references that associate the psalmist's painful condition with his wrongdoing. The sufferer's cry laments his offense and foolishness for the distress they subsequently caused him. The matter of making meaning out of great pain is foregrounded at the outset of Psalm 38. Responses to the why questions of the genesis and purpose of pain appear immediately: pain is the result and deserved punishment for wrongdoing. We read no defense of innocence, no excuse for misdeeds. The psalmist thinks of his suffering as the result of the just punishment of God, not only citing misdeeds but also matching wrongdoing with God's response. Three initial references to God's anger, told with three different terms (translated "wrath," "rage," and "indignation") are answered by three references to the psalmist's wrongdoing, told with three different words (translated "sin," "wrongdoings," and "foolishness"). Introducing this interpretation, we read a desperate request that God desist from punishing the psalmist, hinting at the change that marks this psalm—a facile interpretation accepted, challenged, and surpassed. The psalmist claims that he already has suffered from God's hand, "your arrows have sunk into me, and your hand has come down on me," and simply on account of behaving badly, "my wrongdoings are like a weighty burden," "my wounds stink and rot because of my foolishness." Broken and crushed by the consequences of his bad life choices, the psalmist cries out.

Embedded in these early complaints and in the verses that follow, we find a strikingly detailed description of the psalmist's painful condition. Although the psalmist describes his pain generally, he also adds detail and specificity that is unusual for psalmic descriptions of pain. The psalmist complains of stinking and rotting wounds, a posture twisted and bent, a constant burning sensation, and frantic exhaustion. Nowhere else in the psalms do we find so much explicit detail of a psalmist's painful condition. However, even these evocative descriptions of specific physical symptoms do not total the experience of pain that Psalm 38 tells. The pain is systemic, generally disintegrating and exhausting the psalmist's entire person. The psalmist tells of "no wholeness in my bones/self," the sense of carrying a heavy burden, and of being "numbed and crushed." The pain is devastating, affecting all aspects of the sufferer, physical, mental, spiritual, and social. Descriptions of the psalmist's painful physical condition are interwoven with expressions of its implications psychologically (e.g. "too weighty for me," "I walk around gloomy"), spiritually (e.g. "longing" for God), and socially (e.g. "those closest to me stand far away"). Although the psalmist associates this pain, described in excruciating detail, with earlier wrongdoing, both the description and its development call into question the virtue of such pain. The pain itself is so damaging to the person that any benefit it might have had as corrective punishment is challenged and undermined.

In his article, "Pain and Resistance," Arthur Kleinman records and analyzes an interview with Stella Hoff, "a thirty-one-year-old Ph.D. biochemistry researcher in medicine who has suffered severe pain for four years following a car accident."[7] In her words, we hear a person in great pain wrestling both with the idea that somehow the pain is justified and also that because of its intensity, the pain finally serves no useful purpose and is instead only damaging. Before the accident, Dr. Hoff pushed herself very hard to succeed in a stressful world of academic research and writing. "Previously I brought all my work home with me. It was bad for my family life and my own peace of mind. I felt driven, and would continue to work late into the night. I felt something tormenting, me, driving me on."[8] She wonders aloud if her doubts about success and anxiety about failing have made of her pain "a disguised form of avoiding failure," though she immediately qualifies this with "I don't think I really believe that, but [. . .]." We hear in her comments this common idea that her pain may be *deserved*, as much by failure (an inability to meet expectations for personal and professional success) as by deliberate wrongdoing. Kleinman observes that attitudes in the late twentieth-century United States among the upper-middle class promoted a "cycle of self-improvement and self-promotion" with a twin "fear of 'falling from grace,'" a kind of "secularized soteriology." Reflecting on Hoff's situation, Kleinman observes, "Not to rise is [. . .] often experienced by members of the American middle class as a shameful moral weakness."[9] Considering personal success in these terms, conditions of pain may be easily interpreted as the logical payment or punishment for failings, simply another way of interpreting pain as deserved punishment.

Psalm 38 demonstrates that such an interpretation need not be the last word; however, but that even when the one in pain claims such meaning for his or her pain, it is possible to think differently about it yet again. It is possible to name the pain as too great, too long, too devastating to be useful. Robert Smith observes, "Most spiritual writers speak of suffering as a school of learning, correction, or advancing wisdom. It follows that the sufferer's own understanding and interpretation of his or her suffering might change over time, and we should not assume that first interpretations are fixed and changeless."[10] While the two requests to God that frame the psalm mark the psalmist's changing interpretation, there is a hint of this change already in the first stanzas, which describe in startling detail the nature of the psalmist's pain. "There is no soundness in my flesh," the psalmist complains twice (verses 3 and 7). The first occurrence is followed immediately by "because of your indignation," but the second lacks this explanation. That is, the psalmist first interprets his painful disintegration as due to deserved punishment, but later eschews any interpretation at all, simply noting how the pain disintegrates him. The repetition of "there is no soundness in my flesh" within different contexts, the first of explanation, the second of simple complaint hints at the psalm's shift from justified pain to justification for relief from such pain. Already within the first part of the psalm, the psalmist's ideas about his pain begin to change, reflecting a sense that the pain is not useful as justified punishment; it has instead become only burdensome and problematic.

As descriptions of a deeply painful condition continue to pile up, reasons become irrelevant. After the first few verses linking pain to wrongdoing, we read details of the painful condition without any accompanying explanation. "I howl from the groaning of my heart [. . .] My mind reels, my strength fails me." The pain is sustained long after determining any meaning for it until, exhausted, the psalmist exclaims, in a suggestively aborted complaint, "the light of my eyes, even they—there is nothing with me." Besides the poignant sense of this clause, its structure demonstrates the fracturing effect of his pain. The psalmist is unable to finish the sentence, to fill out the explanation. The pain is nothing but destructive, finally rendering him unable even to hear and speak. As the psalmist evocatively describes his painful condition, we witness how the psalmist's initial explanation of suffering for wrongdoing gives way simply to complaint of a pain that affects all aspects of his self, broken into pieces, each of which is subject to torment.

The complaint, "there is nothing with me," underscores the sense of being deaf and mute and so hints at the psalmist's social condition of loneliness and rejection. Indeed, not only does the pain wreck him physically, mentally, and spiritually, but it does so in part also socially, straining and breaking relationships with others. The psalmist complains of relationships marked by distance and distrust on account of his pain. "My lovers and friends stand aloof from my injury; those closest to me stand far away." The sparseness of these lines deepens their poignancy, and the juxtaposition of antonyms in the second clause emphasizes the sense that those who would/should be closest to the psalmist are distant. At the center is the word translated, "my injury." The vocabulary and structure of these lines demonstrate how the psalmist's painful condition becomes a central issue between himself and others, making even those who are defined by their proximity and care for the psalmist distant from him, unable and/or unwilling to help.

Again, Stella Hoff's experience with great and persistent pain is instructive. Kleinman observes in the range of Hoff's pain "a particularizing social course of illness experience that is inimical to the biomedical claim of a natural course that unfolds from the disease process itself."[11] Dr. Hoff's pain has immediate and deleterious effects on all of her relationships. The medical professionals who have worked to address her pain express frustration and exasperation, call her "a problem patient [. . .] extremely demanding, and she doesn't get better." Of them, Hoff says, "Pain is too much for physicians to deal with [. . .]. Pain patients like me are a sign of the failure of the medical care system, of something terribly wrong at the core."[12] Like Hoff, many pain patients find that as time goes on without positive results from different diagnoses and treatments, they lose credibility with their caretakers and experience terrific strain on all relationships. Even immediate family relationships are strained. Hoff says, "Now, they [her family] get pretty angry at me. They simply don't understand what is going on."[13]

The sense that those who should be closest to the person in pain have become distant exacerbates the painful condition with loneliness and rejection. The distance of family and friends also may exacerbate already strained relationships between the pained person and his or her caregivers insofar as family and friends advocate less, if at all, for the person in pain. Immediately following complaint about the distance of "those closest to me," the psalmist complains of people whom the psalmist thinks desire to hurt or even kill him. Perhaps these lines describe a real condition of physical threat by others; but maybe the psalmist's perception of his pain is not only the cause of distance from family and friends but is also a source of antagonism toward others. For one thing, other people have trouble understanding chronic pain that is not immediately evident and resists satisfactory diagnosis and treatment. Sometimes such pain is dismissed as an unreal fabrication, creating a vicious cycle as sufferers find it necessary to dramatize their pain, consequently raising questions among their caregivers about the kind of and extent of the pain. The result is a "poisoned clinical atmosphere in which trust and support — so central to the healing process — are replaced by suspicion, accusation, and ultimately a pervasive, mutually frustrating resentment."[14] The psalmist cries out, "I am ready to stumble, my pain is continually before me"; and "many people wrongly hate me [. . .] they harass me instead of trying to do good."

For the person suffering intractable pain, the only possible language, at times, is complaint; but such complaint frequently yields nothing but grief, in part because of how it repels others. Then, silence. In the context of his great pain, the psalmist says, "I am like the deaf, I do not hear; and like the dumb, I do not open my mouth." Hoff explains, "I get angry with myself, but I can't express it, never could. I get very quiet, others learn to leave me alone—thus, I don't address it."[15] Complaint and silence both adversely affect the pained person's relationships to others. The pained person's behavior may be difficult, even toxic, for those close to him; and their reactions are off-putting to the pained person who then may grow angry at or suspicious of them. Kleinman describes Hoff as "distant, formal, even cold in her bearing." He notes a striking intensity about her, which he attributes to "her pain—constant, severe, dominating. Hoff is fighting each moment to remain in control." Psychological testing revealed her experiences of "anxiety, irritability, and fear [. . .] rage, [. . .] and a strong suspiciousness that others treated her badly, could not be trusted, and would take advantage of her if she did not exercise vigilance."[16] The psalmist reiterates that he is not blameless, but reasons that God should nevertheless attend, come near and help, because the psalmist has already suffered pain and sorrow for earlier sin and now also faces the cruelty of others.

The pain is not (or is no longer) useful or even appropriate, the psalmist suggests. It is not doing any good; on the contrary. Hoff says to Kleinman, "Suffering is an evil. I mean suffering that has no meaning, that brings nothing good with it. There is a spiritual side of my pain. That is what I mean by evil. My spirit is hurt, wounded."[17] The psalmist's final request is that God be near, help, and save from a condition in which there is nothing redeeming. In this request, we witness the psalmist's sense that justified or not, his pain has itself become an evil; from it, the psalmist reasons, God ought to save him. The psalm concludes with this prayer, an expression of confidence that no matter his earlier wrongdoings, the psalmist is justified in calling to God for nearness and help simply because "I am ready to collapse; my pain is always with me."

A Wider Lens Affects the View

The internal shift of Psalm 38 from justified pain to self-justification is underscored by a similar move within the greater literary context of Psalms 32–41. Psalm 38's greater literary context supposes that interpretation of one's pain as deserved punishment may be appropriate; but it need not be the last word. Great and lasting pain has devastating effects, personally and socially, that undermine the value of such an interpretation. Interpreting pain as deserved punishment risks reducing a person to no more than his or her sin and its deserved painful punishment, and reducing God to no more than a record-tallying judge. A person who cries out of great pain for help professes to be a whole person, valuably capable of a wide variety of attitudes and actions. Furthermore, he or she witnesses to a God who is radically free to make possible the expression of such personal potential by relieving pain, even pain initially interpreted as just punishment. The psalms that precede and follow Psalm 38 highlight the development within Psalm 38 from interpretation of the psalmist's pain as justified punishment to detailed description of the devastating effects of his or her pain that finally justifies the psalmist's plea for help and mercy.

Although the one or two psalms immediately preceding and following the one in question are its most powerful context by nature of their proximity, I consider the greater literary context of Psalm 38 as it bears on our understanding of that psalm, to include Psalms 32–41. Psalm 32 commends itself as the beginning of Psalm 38's greater literary context partly because Psalm 32 is also a confessional psalm wherein the speaker admits guilt, associates suffering with that condition, and asks God's forgiveness. Because Psalms 32 and 38 share together with Psalms 6, 51, 102, 130, and 143 common characteristics of repentance and hope for forgiveness, these seven psalms come to be known in later Christian tradition as the "Penitential Psalms." I conclude with Psalm 41 partly because it, too, expresses the idea of repentance as critical to health and healing and because it is the last psalm of the first of five groupings in the book of Psalms. However, these are not the only reasons to take into account this greater context of Psalm 38. The manner in which shared images, vocabulary, and ideas appear in Psalms 32–41 informs and affects our understanding and interpretation of Psalm 38, especially concerning both the psalmist's experience of pain and our attempts to make meaning of such pain.

Reading Psalm 38 independent of its context, we sympathize with the psalmist, who admits wrongdoing and seems to suffer disproportionately and continually despite confession of guilt and remorse. The description of the psalmist's tortured physical, psychological, spiritual, and social condition is vivid and arresting. We are "on the psalmist's side." Reading Psalm 38 within the broader context of the psalms preceding and following it, under-cuts and reshapes an impression otherwise based only on Psalm 38. Considered with the psalms preceding it, the psalmist's guilt situates him *in the company of wrongdoers*, so starkly distinguished from the righteous speakers of the immediately preceding psalms. The author of Psalm 38 is admittedly guilty, and by the theological reasoning of the preceding psalms, precisely among those whose distress is justified by their wrongdoing. In those other psalms, such a person is frequently portrayed as the enemy, and his or her pain is a welcome expression of justice understood as God's doing to "right" wrongs and prevent further abuses from happening. The clear distinction between the right-eous and the guilty, each getting their just desserts from God, is strongly represented both in the psalms immedi-ately preceding (Psalms 36–37) and also throughout the greater context (especially in Psalm 34).

Psalm 37, contextually setting the stage for Psalm 38, is spoken by one who counts herself among the innocent and describes a clear distinction between the wicked and the righteous. Its introductory lines leave no doubt that those who do wrong are "the others," by contrast to the speaker and the speaker's community. The author of Psalm 37 declares a comforting confidence that "we, the right," and "they, the wrong" will each get from God just desserts. The voice is that of a wise teacher, counseling patience among his or her community in the certainty that God looks out for those who do right: "I was young, but indeed am now old; yet I have not seen the righteous abandoned nor their children beg for food." The tone is sure that those who do not do right will experience the pain of pun-ishment, even destruction: "transgressors will be totally destroyed, the remainder of the wicked ones cut off." This is a welcome message for those who consider themselves righteous; but for the psalmist of Psalm 38, one wonders. Admittedly, the wicked ones in Psalm 37 are primarily defined in light of relationships to other people, willfully hurting others by physical attack, financial wrongdoing, and oppression, while the crime of the speaker of Psalm 38 is identified only in light of his relationship to God. Nevertheless, many texts describe wrongs against God as wrongs against others.

Coming as it does immediately following Psalm 37, we may read with less sympathy the suffering of the poet of Psalm 38. After all, he admits to wrongdoing, and by the logic of Psalm 37, his suffering is deserved. However, we have seen that Psalm 38 itself shifts in sense from the psalmist's pain as justified punishment by God for the psalmist's wrongdoing to self-justification in the face of both the extraordinary degree of his suffering and the nastiness of others. This self-justification is underscored by the psalm immediately following Psalm 38. Therefore, reading Psalm 38 together not only with what precedes but also what follows confirms our ambivalence about the psalmist. While Psalm 37 suggests that the psalmist's pain is indeed the deserved suffering of a sinner, Psalm 39 strengthens our sense that the psalmist is justified in asking for relief. Psalm 39, closely linked to Psalm 38 in language and sense as well as textual location, deepens our sympathy for the psalmists of both psalms. Psalm 39 represents the words of one who has done wrong but claims to have suffered even more for her silence and demands reprieve from God on account of being simply "human."

The greater context reinforces these observations. There is a clear distinction between the innocent and the guilty with a sense that they accordingly are or will be

rewarded or punished by God; but there is also reference
to suffering that does not fit this clear tit-for-tat theology.
Concerning the latter, we read in these psalms not only
that sometimes the righteous suffer but also that sometimes God should (and does) help those whose suffering is
understood as punishment for their wrongdoing. I have
briefly noted how Psalm 39 picks up on this matter from
Psalm 38. So, too, Psalm 40 heightens the ambivalence
about how to interpret and so handle suffering. Nearly
everything about Psalm 40 portrays the psalmist as righteous—from the psalmist's testimony of God's saving
action on his or her behalf, to recounting how the psalmist
preached God's power and goodness, to being the victim
of the hurt of malicious others. However, without seeming
to challenge this singular impression of the psalmist as a
person of God and deserving of help, the psalmist says of
present suffering, "my iniquities have overtaken me, until
I cannot see; they are more than the hairs of my head, and
my heart fails me." We will reconsider the implications of
these observations after noting some of the characteristics
that link Psalms 32–41 together. Noting and considering
such characteristics may help us make sense of opposing
interpretations of the experience of pain.

The matter of speech, or more accurately keeping silent
versus speaking out, runs through this group of psalms
like a narrow brook. At times it bubbles with speech, the
intention of speaking one's repentance. At times it promotes silence, restraint from speaking what is wrong. At
times, the psalmists express numb silence in the face of
others' wrongdoing; and at times they exuberantly declare
intent to proclaim what is right and good. In Psalm 32,
keeping silent was a bad thing. The psalmist claimed an
early silence, broken finally by determination to repent,

after which she experienced healing. By contrast, it is the pressure of others that renders the author of Psalm 38 mute (not refusal to confess his wrongdoing). Perhaps this is related to the advice of the author of Psalm 33 who says, "keep your tongue from evil and your lips from speaking deceit." Psalm 39 begins with reference to such silence, but claims that such silence only exacerbated her suffering; and subsequent silence reflects resignation that the pain is God's doing and too much to bear. By contrast, Psalm 40 emphasizes speech, especially testimony of God's help. There, the psalmist refers to telling God's saving action no less than eight times [. . .] but does not claim to be without suffering, including a call for deliverance and concluding, "I am poor and needy." The matter of speech and silence runs throughout Psalms 32–41, but it does so in different ways that considered together guide development from justified pain to self-justification and reinforce ambivalence about the meaning for/of pain.

Psalm 34 does not deny that the righteous suffer, but it does express confidence that God helps. Psalm 35 is like Psalm 69 in its identification of hurtful others and a desire for a particular kind of vengeance. Psalm 36 draws a distinction between the wicked and the righteous; Psalm 37 answers with "do not fret because of the wicked," trust, wait, "I am old yet I have not seen the righteous forsaken." Psalm 38 is different. Preceding psalms presume that the ones telling them are among the righteous, not the wicked, in clear dualism. By contrast, the speaker of Psalm 38 is neither clearly righteous nor clearly wicked, neither wholly responsible for his pain nor wholly innocent either. In Psalm 38, the author is rather a God-fearing person who has nevertheless done wrong (we are not told specifically what) and out of a punishing condition seeks help and relief.

Psalm 39 is clearly to be associated with Psalm 38 as its particular vocabulary, point of view, and general content indicate; yet in it the speaker is no miserable wretch but speaks out with dignified anger and expectation of help and relief from God. Rather than concluding with a request that God be near, as in Psalm 38, the author of Psalm 39 concludes with a request that God "look away." Psalm 40 seems to pick up immediately from Psalm 39, yet reflects a change of condition: "I put my hope in YHWH; he leaned toward me, and heeded my cry." The psalmist claims not to have withheld words about God's saving action, loyalty, and love, and then changes to explain a miserable condition and hope for help from God.

The final psalm of this first collection in the book of Psalms is Psalm 41. Its position concluding the group of psalms that we have just considered has powerful implications. Following the debated matters of innocence and guilt, of reward and punishment; following the dismissal of easy justification for pain simply as punishment; and following complaints of utterly unjustified pain, Psalm 41 focuses on how other people treat the person in pain. It is sung in praise of the person who did not hesitate to help the one in trouble. It draws attention to interpersonal relationships in the context of suffering, focusing on the role of other people in (the relief of) a person's pain [. . .] even the pain of a person who has done wrong. Taken together, Psalms 32–41 not only validate the struggle to balance justified punishment with merciful restraint, but they also transcend this issue by elevating and applauding those who help people in pain, whatever the pain's reason. These psalms do not make pain only God's issue but a powerfully social concern, too; and this is the final word of the collection.

A "Tyranny of Meaning"? [18]

Psalm 38, which begins with meaning—the meaning of the psalmist's pain wrapped up in the wrongdoing of which he's guilty—ends simply with an expression of desire that God be near to help and save. We observed in the preceding chapter how Psalm 69 "stays with" the matter of meaning, although it shifts from the meaning *of* one's suffering (reasons for it) to the meaning *for* one's suffering (purpose for it). By contrast, Psalm 38 abandons the matter of justified suffering for description of the psalmist's painful condition, which includes his place vis-à-vis others, and concentrates simply on request for God's presence, proximity, and help. In the process, Psalm 38 questions the necessity and usefulness of establishing meaning for and/or in pain, particularly in the case of justifying the pain as punishment. Robert Smith, a Roman Catholic priest, writes, "The possible meanings of pain are so many, and the reality of suffering in a person's life so complex, that reducing all of this to a single cause as punishment seems simplistic. It may be psychologically understandable as a first reaction, but it betrays the human richness of religious beliefs, and seems to most religious people to imply a grotesque misunderstanding of God."[19] Indeed, such interpretations can also be damaging, even destructive.[20]

Arthur Kleinman criticizes his anthropologist predecessors of a kind of "tyranny of meaning that overvalues coherence and other intellectualist priorities at the expense of everything else [. . .]."[21] He notes, "The literary imagination's revulsion against, and the popular culture's reaction to, the bloody havoc of our century has challenged the dominion of meaning as inadequate, distorting, or even inhuman."[22] Kleinman appeals to the

voices especially of Holocaust survivors for eloquent and
poignant reminders that assigning meaning to and for suffering is not always possible and sometimes causes a great
deal more pain. Kleinman observes, "the absolute primacy
of concern with meaning—meaning that is understood as
a cognitive response to the challenge of coherence—
would seem to be dubious. [. . .] It places greater value on
'knowing the world,' as William James put it, than on
inhabiting, acting in, or wrestling with the world."[23]

Although the psalmist interprets his own pain and so
does not demonstrate the problematic nature of interpreting another's pain for him or her, it reflects both the manner in which cultural characteristics of thinking influence
the individual's and how others' interpretation of one's
own pain can exacerbate it. Meaning-making can be con-
scripted into a jockeying for power as "a political tool that
reworks experience so that it conforms to the demands of
power."[24] That is, if meaning-making happens "from
above," rather than with the one(s) suffering, then the one
actually suffering loses his or her voice. The ones suffering
are then reduced to silence and objectified in a manner
that strips the sufferer of agency and self-determination.
Finding others malicious and treacherous, the psalmist
exclaims, in a sense, "in the meaning-making of others, I
am rendered deaf and mute."

Susan Sontag has drawn criticism for her attempt to
resist metaphoric ways of thinking about illness, the goal
she states for her book *Illness as Metaphor*. She explains,
"the most truthful way of regarding illness—and the
healthiest way of being ill—is one most purified of, most
resistant to, metaphoric thinking."[25] I, too, find this problematic in light of the fact that a person might communicate suffering effectively through simile and metaphor.
However, Sontag seems to be concerned most with exag-

gerating the difficult mysteries about illness in a way that compromises a patient's attitude and approach to his or her illness. This contributes something to our understanding of the psalmist's wrestling in Psalm 38 insofar as the application of meaning may compromise one's ability to manage the very real pain for what it is. Sometimes the search for meaning is itself problematic. The psalmist admits wrongdoing and accepts that one way to interpret his suffering is as divine punishment for this behavior. However, the psalmist does not end there; rather, he argues for life beyond such "tyranny of meaning," for relief *anyway*. The psalmist is bigger and more multifaceted than his previous actions and even than his pain; and in the condition of pain, the psalmist exclaims, "I am worthy—of right treatment by others, even of the presence and succor of God." George Herbert wrote a poem loosely based on Psalm 38 titled "Complaining," in which he challenges the reduction of a pained person only to his or her suffering and the reduction of God only to justice. "Art thou all justice, Lord? / Shows not thy word / More attributes? Am I all throat or eye, / To weep or cry? / Have I no parts but those in grief?"

It would seem that Sontag argues against a kind of meaning-making with metaphors that finally and paradoxically ignores the actual illness and that critically comments on the sufferer in a way that denies him or her the dignity of coming to terms with the reality of his or her condition. The psalmist does not suddenly argue that he is innocent, but rather that guilt need not have anything to do with his pain [. . .] or with its relief. Out of destructive pain, the psalmist asserts the legitimacy of mercy, *simply as a human being* asking for God's attention and help. By its end, the psalm is "more about the expression of suffering than the meaning behind it, more about the vicissitudes of survival than the abstractions of sin and guilt, and more about *protest* as a religious posture than capitulation or confession."[26] For the person who interprets his or her pain as the just punishment of God for some wrongdoing, Psalm 38 may provide a companion that takes such thinking seriously but does not end there. In protesting against it, in criticizing the failure of others to be "for" the psalmist, and in boldly asking for God's nearness and help, the psalmist demonstrates a sense of dignity and self-worth that transcends the tyranny of meaning and justifies relief. The psalmist both admits wrongdoing and calls into question the role of an absolute justice that tortures and destroys the one who did wrong.

Reading the psalm, we witness a manner of interpreting and living through one's pain that is sensible both for an individual's experience of his or her pain and for those who take care of someone who interprets his or her pain in this manner. Psalm 38 reflects the interpretation of one's own pain; it is told from the perspective of the one suffering. In the process of listening to it, we are invited to be a "someone else" who attends to the psalmist's interpretation, is present through the psalmist's process of challenging such an interpretation, and finally can appreciate the psalmist as a person justified in desiring relief from his or her pain. Psalm 38 warns readers both against interpreting another's pain and against prematurely "correcting" interpretations that may seem inappropriately damning. Instead, it takes seriously the possibility that a person may initially interpret his or her pain as justified punishment for wrongdoing; but it challenges holding on to such an interpretation in the face of pain's destructive power.

Psalm 38 is told from the perspective of the one suffering and so reflects the interpretation by the one in pain of his or her own pain. Reading Psalm 38 gives us occasion to think about the role of an interpretation of pain that declares that pain is the deserved punishment for wrong-doing, the place of such an interpretation, and justification for challenging it. Reading Psalm 38 invites us to consider how such an interpretation may yield to the legitimacy of mercy if for no other reason than that reasons are overridden by the extent and duration of the pain itself. The ideas expressed in Psalm 38 are dynamic, and in this process of change, readers witness a simple interpretation accepted, challenged, and demoted. Psalm 38 offers us an opportunity to consider critically the interpretation of pain as punishment or payment for some kind of wrongdoing or debt and how any such interpretation may finally be less relevant than the pain that is suffered insofar as such pain, destructive of the whole person, legitimates mercy. A pain that fractures a person and destroys relationships is useless at best. Psalm 38 tells that anyone, no matter who or how, is justified in seeking support and relief in the face of dehumanizing pain. Psalm 38 testifies to the place of mercy in human affairs simply because of being human.

6

Finally Darkness (Psalm 88)

✑

*"My self is full of troubles, my life is on the brink
of the land of the dead."*

The struggle between justice and mercy, between a
"relentlessly contractual" theology and the protest against
it, between sense and non-sense, is at play in the paradoxical nature of making meaning out of chronic pain. Both of
the psalms that we have already considered, Psalms 69
and 38, demonstrate efforts to understand the pain, to
interpret the meaning behind it and purpose for it. That
such efforts may not finally yield definitive answers and
may even complicate and compound the experience of
pain illustrates the "tyranny of meaning" that we considered in the preceding chapter.

Psalm 88 is the sustained cry of a person whose pain
feels fatal. She is desperate and lonely, and the pain she
suffers is not explained as the result of the psalmist's or
anyone else's actions. In Psalm 88, there is no mention of
what the psalmist may have done or not done to explain
her pain. Although it mentions the anger of God, nowhere
do we read of the psalmist's sin as the reason for God's
anger and punishment like we did in Psalm 38. Furthermore, there is no sense that antagonism, threat, or attack

by others lies behind the psalmist's pain. Although we read of a loneliness that exacerbates the psalmist's pain, we do not find reference to enemies who cause or exacerbate the pain, like we did in Psalm 69. Instead, God alone is the cause, and there seems to be no good reason for it. Psalm 88 is dark. In what follows, I briefly discuss the psalm in general, as a candid yet eloquent expression of the feeling of deepest dark despair that intractable pain can elicit. I then consider more specifically the presence and role of anger in Psalm 88 and in experiences of pain. This includes both the psalmist's anger and the anger of God. Finally, I address the matter of darkness as the psalm's conclusion, considering the different ways that we might understand it and the intriguing implications it has for the experience of pain.

"Pain—Has an Element of Blank" [1]

Psalm 88 is unique among the book of Psalms for its persistent complaint. It does not include the expressions of thanksgiving or even of hope that other psalms do. Instead, the psalmist begins with complaint and ends with darkness. In between, there seems to be no discernible progress; rather, we are confronted with the bitter fact that the psalmist's pain and near-death condition, with its attendant loneliness and sense of abandonment by God, is the sum total. Lacking "coherent sequence" and "discernible causality," Psalm 88 shares characteristics with what Arthur Frank calls a "chaos narrative" in which "troubles go all the way down to the bottomless depths."[2] Any description of such a condition is a series of disconnected fragments of complaint, not a sensible story with progressive development. This is the expression out of frustration and despair that, if it can be articulated at all, is anguished complaint with no real beginning and no clear end. It lacks any sense of looking forward to better times, with restitution of health and/or happiness.

It is tempting for others to identify in such a condition of dark despair the possibility, even promise, of personal growth, renewal, and restoration to conditions better than before precisely because of enduring such difficulty. The popularity of Nietzche's "what does not kill you makes you stronger" attitude is testimony to that. Indeed, looking back on such dark times, occasionally people conclude that something good came from them — new opportunities and insights, maybe an important period of personal growth. However, that is not always the case (and never appropriate to claim about someone else's pain), and such conclusions are possible only after looking back on them. In the context of the experience itself, in the deepest darkest time, suffering may seem to be all that there is, and the possibility of a better future is meaningless. This is the condition Marni Jackson associates with four A.M., a time after the "hopeful" hours before midnight and the "mild drama" and "sense of a solitary tryst with the self" that are possible between one and two A.M. yet still before the dawn. The predawn hours, worst around four o'clock, "are scary, bottomless hours, [. . .] like a dog with a bone, pain runs away with you."[3]

The present darkness is all there is and seems to be all there ever will be. Emily Dickinson writes, "Pain — has an Element of Blank —," an idea that she develops in this poem as the sense of pain erasing memory of any time before the pain and of no future except pain.[4] Any movement out of such a condition is by definition not-yet; it is not the sufferer's present reality. Only the darkness, only the despair is real and present for such a person. It is important, then, to recognize this and to refrain from pushing into hope and relief that may simply not be, at that time, within the sufferer's scope of possibility. "The worst thing medical staff can do to someone in the chaos story is rush him to move on. Moving on is desirable; chaos is the pit of narrative wreckage. But attempting to push the person out of this wreckage only denies what is being experienced and compounds the chaos."[5]

We spend some time with Psalm 88 at this point in the book because it presses us to accept the bitter reality that any movement *out of* a condition of darkest despair and anything positive that may come of it supposes the experience *of* such a condition. The condition that Psalm 88 expresses is real precisely because it is without false hope or premature thanksgiving. It is simply an honest cry of darkest despair. "The challenge of encountering the chaos narrative is how not to steer the storyteller away from her feelings. [. . .] The challenge is to hear."[6] We meditate on Psalm 88 as the midpoint in our contemplation of half a dozen psalms partly because it tells the nadir of pain. Our reading of it, at this point, follows our reading of struggles for meaning and complaint concerning the particular, debilitating conditions that we read in Psalms 38 and 69; and it comes before our study of psalms that reflect (again) hope and even thanksgiving. Not everyone experiences the dark night that Psalm 88 tells, but for those who do it can be devastating. This thorny and difficult psalm acknowledges that sometimes in the experience of great and lasting pain, there is this anguish and seemingly only that. We do well to settle in to this uncomfortable psalm and allow it its voice without anticipating what it does not express—better times ahead.

Like the soil of my Virginia garden in the fall after a long stretch of rainy days, this psalm is black and saturated. It hints of rot. But while the soil is full of water, the psalm is full of grief, despair, and complaint. The psalmist complains that her very self, *nephesh*, is filled with troubles and has been since childhood. This Hebrew term, *nephesh*, which I briefly defined above, captures the sense that Teresa of Avila and John of the Cross mean by the Spanish *alma*, "soul." Reflecting on the writings of these sixteenth-century mystics, Gerald May explains, "When Teresa and John speak of the soul, they are not talking about something a person *has*, but who a person most deeply *is*: the essential spiritual nature of a human being."[7] In Psalm 88, the poet complains that who she is, is saturated by troubles. When nephesh appears again in the psalm, it is with fists flailing at the gates of heaven: "Why, God, do you spurn my very self?"

In the psalmist's condition of trouble and abandonment, death stands gaping. The psalmist cries out that her life is on the edge of death, "on the brink of Sheol." Within just a few verses (4-6), the psalmist four times situates herself in the grave, already counted a resident of the place of the dead. Emily Dickinson writes, "Pain has but one Acquaintance / And that is Death –."[8] Indeed, the psalmist claims that death has been with her since childhood: "I am afflicted and close to death from my youth." Death is a dominant presence in the psalm with many and diverse references: *sheol*, the pit, the grave, the place of ruin, the land of oblivion, and darkness. That death is ever-present to this speaker in great pain contributes to her sense of terrible loneliness—loss of human companionship as well as abandonment by God. Indeed the seeming complicity and silence of God is inseparable from the psalmist's pain, and the sense that others have consigned her to death exacerbates the fear and despair.

In our times of medical "miracles," a human life may be prolonged far past the point that the individual wishes, past the point that the individual feels capable of being who he or she is and feels instead to be a burden that others have dismissed for dead. Although this psalm was composed when the life span of any person was short by today's standards, it speaks to many whose suffering goes on and on. It speaks to those whose condition feels fatal, but lingers in a torturous state. Worn down by pain, life is full of trouble, terror, and the anticipation of more of the same suffering. Seemingly near death, such people find in the behavior of others a sense that they have already been given up for dead. I am reminded of an independent woman in her 80s who lived in the same apartment building as I did in Boston. We became friends. She told me colorful stories of her adventures as a socialite and traveler. One afternoon she returned from a doctor's appointment very upset. She had expressed concern about spots on her hands, not only that they may represent an early skin cancer but also that they were ugly to her. Her doctor told her that it wasn't worth treating them; she probably would not live much longer than ten years more, anyway. She was devastated—"counted among those going down to the Pit" and dismissed from human sympathy.

Anatole Broyard said that he wanted "to make sure I'll be alive when I die" and wrote of the necessity that each person develop "a style" for their dying, that every one die in keeping with who and how he or she is.[9] Intractable pain complicates things. We all want to die reconciled with family and friends and comfortable in our relation to God, but pain gets in the way. Pain complicates such a death in several ways. The sufferer's essence seems saturated by trouble; consequently, he or she may feel that "I'm not myself," yet also be unable to reconstruct that self. Furthermore, those closest to the sufferer may pull away, abruptly or gradually, relating differently if at all to the difficult person that pain makes of him or her. And pain may make God seem distant or willfully disinterested in a person's plight. Prayers for help and relief yield neither, and the sufferer's faith brings no comfort, if it lasts at all. Psalm 88 is an honest cry out of such a condition. Its inclusion in the Bible dignifies the terror, anxiety, loneliness, and despair that may characterize significant periods of days, weeks, months, maybe years in the life of a person suffering intractable pain.

By contrast to the other psalms that we consider here, Psalm 88 is addressed entirely to God. Its sustained attention on God, choice of address or name for God, and the content of its prayer demonstrate a deep personal relationship and enduring desire for God. That God is silent makes the psalm particularly poignant. The psalmist's first word is the divine name: that is, the psalmist begins by addressing God with the personal name, YHWH, that denotes God's special relationship with a particular people. At the root of this four-letter name is the verb "to be." Consequently, the name, YHWH, *HaShem*, the LORD declares that this is the God who *is*, will be, and brings into being. By beginning with this word, then, the psalmist boldly proclaims a personal relationship with the God who is. The psalmist begins with a confession of faith in the God who is, and   is personally, intimately, covenantally bound to the psalmist's people. Then the psalmist boldly continues by identifying this one as "God of my salvation." It is an auspicious beginning—gutsy in its claims, direct in its address.

With such an address, the psalmist immediately hints at a critical paradox. Following the introductory reference that neatly tells of the psalmist's special relationship (personal, and bound by promise to the psalmist's people) to a God who is defined by existence, by being, the psalmist complains that she is ignored and threatened with death by this very God. The psalmist exclaims that she has consistently and persistently called out to God; yet God seems not to grant the psalmist a hearing. As the psalm continues, so does this problem: "I cry for help to you, O YHWH; in the morning my prayer greets you. Why do you reject me, why hide yourself from me?" Indeed, pain frequently elicits great desire for God's attention and presence, frustratingly simultaneous with a sense of God's silence and seeming absence.

The poet of Psalm 88 takes this relationship further, though, arguing that God should carefully consider how nice it is to have the psalmist's attention before consigning her to a death that prohibits such praise and good publicity. This may seem odd, even preposterous to us. The psalmist presumes that she is important to God, that God actually needs the attention that the psalmist gives and no one else can satisfy this need. Of all the other people in the world, or even simply within the psalmist's community, the psalmist assumes that God would lose out by allowing her, in all of her particularity, to die at this time. There is no question whether or not the psalmist's part in worship is crucial to God's self-interest. Instead, there is an implicit assumption that God would care deeply and suffer a notable loss if the psalmist were to die and so cease telling of God's greatness and good works.

Although there are other ideas about death represented within both the Old and New Testaments, ideas that attest to a relationship with God that continues after death, Psalm 88 reflects an ancient idea that death marked the end of such a relationship. No matter how a person lives, according to this thinking, everyone goes to the same place after death, and it is a place markedly separate from God. The psalmist presumes that out of self-interest in the psalmist's praise and witness to God's goodness, God would come to her aid now, if for no other reason than to preserve a voice of praise and promotion. The psalm is disarmingly honest. To assume that one knows what God wants and actually tell God by way of reminder is nothing less than incredible. Yet in the psalmist's pain, we hear expressions of great intimacy; and in a condition of persistent silence from God, the psalmist is not reluctant to issue presumptuous claims. Considering such attitudes and remarks in the context of the psalm's ending suggests that they may not be so misplaced, after all.

Finally, following a description of the psalmist's terrible condition as the doing of God, a doing that overwhelms the psalmist like floodwaters sweeping down, the psalmist concludes that God also has distanced those who should be closest to the psalmist and so also cut off the comfort and support that they might provide to the sufferer. The psalmist, then, seemingly has "gone nowhere" in the course of this psalm. Complaints of God's ignoring, rejecting, and/or hiding from the sufferer in her pain and distress are combined with descriptions of the sense of being overwhelmed by trouble and terribly alone, drowning in pain and distanced from friends and family. The psalm's last word is "darkness." In light of that, it is remarkable that throughout the psalm, the psalmist's attention is unfailingly on God. This is not insignificant, with implications both for how we understand the place and role of anger in the psalm and also for how we understand the reference to darkness that concludes it.

Sometimes Anger is Infuriating

There is considerable anger in Psalm 88. The psalmist claims that God's anger is at the heart of her suffering; and the psalmist is angry at God. The psalmist's frustration at

God's inattention seems to rise and fall in waves of anger and despair. A significant component in Psalm 88, this anger makes modern readers uncomfortable. Most of us are taught to curb our anger, hide it, or better yet, not to feel angry at all. The idea of God's anger also has been dismissed by people today, ignored or explained away as an antiquated, prescientific understanding of catastrophe. Some see it as an Old Testament notion overridden by better understandings of social and scientific phenomena and/or Jesus' New Testament emphasis on love. Much is wrong about these simplistic reductions. In order to understand and appreciate anger's part in the chaos narrative of Psalm 88, it is important first to accept that there is precedent not only for the place and role of God's anger in the Bible, but also for believing that anger has a place among people, too—even "God's people."

The anger of God is indeed a prominent part of the Hebrew Bible. Bound to God by a covenant that they keep breaking, the Israelites regularly tick God off. Furthermore, we read that God becomes angry at other nations, especially for a pride and arrogance that neglects the sovereignty and power of God. These are general examples of divine anger as justified and its expression necessary. The logic is simple: in order to maintain order, and respect the holiness and sovereignty of God, such anger must be expressed. But there are more subtle aspects, too. Keeping their agreement with God involves people's caring rightly for each other and the world around them. Anger at human neglect or refusal to do so is directly related to the health and well-being of people and the earth. It is important to note, though, that anger is hardly the only facet of God described in the Hebrew Bible. Among many others, mercy, grace, and forgiveness also appear with comforting frequency.

New Testament stories of Jesus reveal that he carried on his faith's tradition of expressing anger at injustice and inhumanity. The most memorable example for many people is the episode of Jesus overturning the moneychangers' tables and throwing them out of the temple. However, the first reference to Jesus' anger has to do with healing. Garrett Keizer notes, "it may be difficult to relocate the theme of healing that lies at the very core of the gospel proclamation without also locating the original anger of Christ."[10] In this episode, Jesus prepares to heal a man's withered hand; but others demand that he wait until the Sabbath is over. Clearly prioritizing human well-being over the letter of the law, Jesus doesn't wait.[11]

"Though we are fully prepared to grant that to forgive is divine, we are a bit reluctant to grant that rage — as opposed to despairing or destroying oneself — can also be divine."[12] Yet human anger, too, has precedent in biblical texts. Moses regularly gets angry with the people in the wilderness and even angry with God for foisting the troublesome lot on him (Numbers 11). We read that David reacted in anger at God for God's killing Uzziah when he steadied the ark (2 Samuel 6) and was rightly angry when he learned that his son Amnon had raped his half-sister Tamar (2 Samuel 13 and 1 Chronicles 13). The prophets are famous for their righteous anger. Amos rails against the wealthy Israelites for taking advantage of the poor and for imagining that their status and possessions reflect God's approval. Malachi gets angry at the Israelite men for divorcing their Jewish wives and so reducing the women to a more vulnerable socio-economic situation, in order to marry foreigners.

In Psalm 88 there is no reason given for God's anger, an anger that the psalmist declares overwhelms her like great waves, yet it seems to be the only reason that the psalmist can conceive of for her pain. The psalmist's unapologetic accusation that God is actually the agent behind the psalmist's miserable condition is striking and discordant to our ears. Great personal suffering and distress is not described in this psalm as due either to personal misbehavior or the machinations of enemies. Instead, God is behind it all, and the psalmist doesn't hesitate to say so, blaming God for her terrible pain. One of the costs of a "radical monotheism," the belief that there is only one supernatural deity, is that everything must be attributed to that One. There is no place for an alter-ego, a devil for example, who can be blamed for what is wrong; rather, God is responsible for everything.[13]

Sometimes it is difficult to reconcile the image of God as the model and basis of all goodness and justice with the image of God as "powers beyond our understanding or control,"observes rabbi and philosophy professor Elliot Dorff. Yet "when the term 'God' denotes the powers that we experience in life beyond our understanding or control, God definitely is involved in undeserved human suffering."[14] Then, "at the extremes of mortal experience, anger at God is not so much a right to be exercised or a problem to be resolved as it is a truth to be lived."[15] Reflecting such thinking, the author of Psalm 88 declares that, even lacking justification or reason for suffering, God is the cause of her pain.

There is no doubt that anger can be destructive, but there is a place for it, too. It is tempting to explain away the anger that colors Psalm 88 as nothing more than the psalmist's desperation and projection; but it is there nonetheless and demands a fuller accounting. There are many references in this psalm to God's anger but no references to the psalmist's deserving to be the object of it.

There is no mention of what the psalmist may have done to provoke or otherwise elicit God's anger, which the psalmist complains lies at the foundation of her distress. The psalmist, too, seems angry—frustrated that God seems to be utterly ignoring her in her plight. The psalmist is angry that God caused such pain, angry that God seems to have forgotten that the psalmist cannot continue to praise God after death, and angry that God pushed away the psalmist's friends and those who loved her. The psalm begins with exasperation, which quickly turns in tone to anger—the psalmist's anger at God.

In an outburst of pent-up accusations, the psalmist says, "you [. . .], you [. . .], you [. . .], you [. . .]" did this to me. No less than four times in a few verses (verses 6-8), with no break in between, the psalmist declares, "you put me [. . .] you overwhelm me, [. . .] you distanced from me [. . .] you set me up." And immediately following this wave of rage, the psalmist deflates, "spent." The psalm moves like the crashing waves it describes, cresting with passionate exclamations, and retreating in exhaustion and supplication. It begins with a white-capped crest—"I cry out to you!"—and then slides into the despairing description of a near-death condition, "overwhelmed with all [God's] breakers." It crests again with the accusation I noted above, and retreats with a single word *spent*. It rises again in a last-ditch attempt to convince God that it is in God's best interest to relieve the psalmist, rescue her from death, and retreats again to reflect on the psalmist's constant but futile attempts to get God's attention. In a final gasp, the psalmist tells of drowning in God's anger, loneliness, and then darkness.

Throughout the psalm, the psalmist's attention on God is unfailing, and this has implications for how we understand the psalmist's anger. Rather than turning away from God, rejecting divine power, care, or even existence, the psalmist persists in her relationship to God. The psalmist's anger, therefore, is not dismissive; on the contrary, it is born of frustration at trying to gain God's hearing and help and of desire for God's presence and attention. It is remarkable that the psalmist does not argue whether or not suffering the anger of God is justified. Instead, it is simply accepted as the source of her pain. God's anger does not seem to be the immediate reason for the psalmist's anger; instead, the *silence* of God infuriates the psalmist. God's distance or willful hiding in the face of the psalmist's great desire for God's attention is cause for the psalmist's frustration and anger. In other words, the psalmist's anger is an anger born of love.

Hello, Darkness — My Old Friend?

After the rise and fall of anger and despair in the face of great pain, the last word of this chaos narrative is darkness. It is a bit of a mystery because the syntax of the line is difficult to discern and the final word itself may mean "darkness" (as "a dark place"), "from darkness," or, least likely, "in darkness."[16] Its mystery and difficulty, however, mirrors its solution, and in the process proposes an understanding of this condition of deepest despair that may be surprising in its implications. That is, there is no one way to read the ending of this psalm any more than there is one way to read the experience of darkness in a context such as Psalm 88's. This has intriguing possibilities for our understanding of the deep darkness, which great and intractable pain may elicit.

That the psalm ends with darkness may in itself be no surprise. Even readers grow exhausted by the psalmist's unrequited cries and chronic condition of being on the edge of death. "Darkness" seems a fitting conclusion to the frustration and despair that unrelieved pain can bring, darkness as metaphor and darkness as the condition in which pain is at its worst. Of the former, we need only to think of the many times depression or hopelessness is described in terms of darkness. People write of "the dark periods" of painters such as Vincent Van Gogh and Francisco Goya, times of great personal distress reflected in paintings dominated by darkness. And things always seem much worse in the dark. "Darkness becomes a cave in which pain swells, until the night feels engorged with it," Marni Jackson writes. "The world outside the circumference of this pain goes blank and becomes unimaginable."[17]

Furthermore, shutting out the sight of others and world outside of oneself, darkness throws the solitary nature of the sufferer into relief. Indeed, unremitting pain is profoundly lonely. In her reflections on the book of Job and speaking out of her own wrestling with pain, biblical scholar Carole Fontaine observes, "those who suffer find their whole world bounded by the experience of their pain. In a very real sense, every sufferer suffers alone and neither talk nor silence blurs that one reality."[18] The psalmist is cut off from the company of others; those who have known and loved the psalmist seem far from him or her. To make matters worse, even God, the one to whom the psalmist has faithfully prayed and whom the psalmist has praised, is unresponsive to her cry for help from great suffering. Such conditions are dark indeed, earning them the label, "dark nights of the soul."

There is another way of thinking about this darkness, however, and we find it represented in the mystical traditions of the one who coined that phrase. It is related to the sense of bleak despair, yet finally results in the

opposite. That is, such darkness is related to the conditions of feeling abandoned, alone, and greatly distressed;
however, John of the Cross with his mentor Teresa of
Avila determined that such periods are characterized by
the mysterious care of God who darkens the senses in
order to enable one to experience a yet more authentic
sense of God. Such periods are difficult indeed, yet they
mark important times of transition to a deepening relationship with God whose love creates darkness as safety
for the soul in its trek to new awakening. Consequently,
John calls such a dark night, *noche que guiaste*, and *noche
amable más que el alborada* ("guiding night," and "night
more lovely than the dawn"). He agrees that the period
seems defined by pain and abandonment by God, and
cites Psalm 88 by way of example. Yet, John writes that
despite such bleak thoughts and feelings, God is actually
even more keenly and closely involved with the sufferer
and is so precisely because the dark makes it possible.
According to John, the light hinders us because we think
we know where we're going. Therefore, "God darkens our
awareness *in order to keep us safe*."[19] And the deepening
darkness is paradoxically indicative of greater divine
light. "For the nearer the soul approaches Him, the
blacker is the darkness which it feels and the deeper is the
obscurity which comes through its weakness; just as the
nearer a man approaches the sun, the greater are the darkness and the affliction caused him through the great splen-
dour of the sun and through the weakness and impurity of
his eyes."[20] Mary Earle, an Episcopal priest who wrote
about applying the Benedictine practice of *lectio divina* to
wrestling with the experience of illness, relates the story
of a woman whose thinking about darkness changed
markedly after meditating on the psalmic text "Darkness

is not dark to you" (Psalm 139:11). Over time, she discovered that her attitude toward a darkness that had haunted her from a traumatic surgical experience changed. Rather than distressing her, the darkness became "welcoming, encompassing, maternal."[21]

That this interpretation of darkness as a hopeful reference may be appropriate at the end of Psalm 88 finds support in the unswerving attention that the psalmist gives to God. We observed above that the psalmist is unapologetic in expressing anger toward God. Such address is impossible without a close relationship. The psalmist reveals an intimacy to God in her accusations of God's *ignoring* her and expressions of personal hurt that God's distance causes. Keizer observes that the domestic context of anger is a powerful one. It is in the company of those who know us best (and maybe love us anyway) that we may "let loose" our feelings of hurt, loss, misunderstanding, and unmet desire. Furthermore, such feelings frequently reflect the depth of love and desire that we have for the one at whom we are angry. That this is the case with the author of Psalm 88 is supported by regular references to deep disappointment and hurt at God's neglect and by frequently reiterated desire for God's attention. These experiences are also indicative of the "dark night of the soul" as described by Teresa of Avila and John of the Cross. Teresa is remembered for saying to Jesus after a particularly painful sense of absence, "If this is how you treat your friends, it is no wonder that you have so few of them." In his *Spiritual Canticle*, John writes of the wounds he suffers from God, his *Amado*, "Beloved" who then fled and hid despite John's searching and calling for God; and Teresa writes of her soul, like a lover, suffering and fainting for desire of God.[22]

Indeed, references of intimate and personal relationship with God run through the psalm, beginning with the first word, the personal name YHWH, and its immediate epithet, "God of my salvation." May observes that the Hebrew term here translated "my salvation" refers to the same "freeing from attachment" that the dark night of the soul accomplishes. "In contrast to life-denying asceticism that advocates freedom *from* desire, Teresa and John see authentic transformation as leading to freedom *for* desire. For them, the essence of all human desire is love."[23] Perhaps the conclusion of Psalm 88 marks entry into a dark night of the soul that is a turning-point of relationship to God. At the psalm's end, the pain and sorrow that dominated preceding verses are scorched by the near light of God. Perhaps we read at the end of Psalm 88 how God satisfies the psalmist's deepest desire and answers the psalmist's repeated requests by entering into a mystical union with him. The psalm moves, then, from the sense of "*oh!*" miserable darkness, to "*ah!*" welcome darkness.

One other matter also supports such an understanding. The psalmist's pestering questions about how God might feel to lose the psalmist's adoration and praise reflect the possibility that contemplatives such as John and Teresa raise that God actually *needs* us, that God is vulnerable. May observes, "Teresa's sense of the Holy One's being surrendered to us in love and *needing* us to love, to be loved by, and to manifest God's love in the world."[24] The thing that most distinguishes such a dark night from depression is the desire especially to love. The psalmist's constant attention to God suggests that even in the context of her great pain, feelings of abandonment by God, and distance from human companions, desire for God, and love for God, continues in the manner that Teresa and John so eloquently describe.

This is surprisingly in keeping with the psalmist's anger at God for turning away and hiding from the psalmist, if we think with Keizer of "anger as an emotion of extreme frustration [. . .] poised at the possibility of action."[25] For the poet of Psalm 88, God is the reason for her great pain—a suffering that reeks with death and is saturated with loneliness and grief. It may be possible to think of the dark night as bringing about a welcome transformation and deeper, more satisfying relationships; but only the suffering person can determine that for himself or herself. Rachel Naomi Remen tells the story of an academic inquiry that yielded unexpected results. In the context of a workshop on Jungian theory and technique, panelists asked participants to respond by standing in silence to "a horrific recurring dream, in which the dreamer was stripped of all human dignity and worth through Nazi atrocities." Asked later to explain their refusal critically to investigate the symbolism and implications, one of the participants said that some suffering is so extreme as to be unspeakable. "In the face of such suffering all we can do is bear witness so no one need suffer alone."[26] Psalm 88 is a companion for those in the dark night that pain can bring. Although its conclusion is ambiguous, its honesty is appealing. Without apology and with great candor, the psalmist dignifies the frustration and anger that a person whose pain is unrelenting and whose loneliness is piercing may feel. The soil of my little garden after days of constant rain smells of rotting things; but by some mystery, somehow, hidden in its darkness, it is also saturated with life.

7

Shared Treasure from a Lonely Journey (Psalm 22)

"For God did not disdain or abhor the affliction of the afflicted nor did God hide God's face from him."

Pain has a social dimension. It is not bounded by the dimensions of a body but is affected by and also affects other people. We have already briefly considered ways in which the psalmist's social context affects his experience of pain, and we will explore this further in reading Psalm 22. Influence goes the other way, too. Pain leaks out like dye to change the color and quality of the pained person's social context. The pained person's experience affects those around him or her, for good and ill, in ever-widening circles, some of which may be beyond his or her view. Psalm 22 invites us to consider this two-way influence in the context of the psalmist's dynamic pain experience.

Reading Psalm 22, we journey with a person through intense pain and loneliness to reintegration into the psalmist's community. The reunion, like the journey, is marked by pain, but it is so by means of what the psalmist's experience can mean for others — by declaration that affliction is not ignored and that help is woven into the fabric of the world. After his own journey through pain and loneliness, the psalmist is able to contribute something uniquely valuable to his community, the voice of one who "knows," and on account of this special knowledge is able both to bring hope and encouragement to others and to be the expression of grace, accepted and integrated as part of the greater community.

Appealing to Joseph Campbell's archetype of the hero helps us to appreciate the arc of Psalm 22 as the psalmist first struggles with an isolating, dehumanizing pain, and then rejoins the community on terms inclusive of the pain experience. After considering the general characteristics and movement of the psalm, I will briefly explain Campbell's theory of the hero's journey and demonstrate the ways in which this archetype illuminates aspects of the psalm's content and movement. In the process, we will also see that, in a crucial way, the psalm challenges Campbell's theory, provoking readers to reconceptualize the notion of hero.

The speaker's social context drives Psalm 22. In the preceding chapter, we considered an aspect of the experience of pain that was utterly introspective and/or focused on God. By contrast to Psalm 88, Psalm 22 is more troubled by and concerned with human exclusion and inclusion than by God's absence. While Psalm 88 decried God's seeming absence or willful ignoring of the psalmist in his pain, Psalm 22 is especially concerned with social rejection; and while Psalm 88 longed for a sense of the presence of God—a longing that the conclusion hints may be satisfied in a kind of mystical union—Psalm 22 anticipates reunion with members of the psalmist's community in recognition of commonality, yet with something unique that the psalmist has to offer others. Unlike Psalm 88, which focuses on God and yearns for restoration of that relationship, Psalm 22 is more human-centered, concerned first with social rejection and isolation and then with reintegration and contribution within the community.

The psalm begins with a description of excruciating pain. It is made so as much by loneliness and social rejection as by any physical condition. Feelings of being less than human and rejected by others contribute as much to the magnitude of distress as does the physical condition itself. A recent study, conducted by John Lunn, Protestant minister and former president of the Kauai Hospice Board of Directors in Hawaii, demonstrates this relationship between social condition and the experience of pain. In the process of working in a hospice program for prisoners, Lunn discovered that inmates would rather suffer greater pain than isolation. To guard against the unauthorized sale of pain medications, prisoners administered such medications are kept isolated in the infirmary. Lunn observed, "given the choice of improved pain control in the infirmary or remaining in their dorm, they always chose the dorm—despite poorer pain control on the physical level."[1] The psalmist's pain has an added level of social complication. Unlike the prisoners of Lunn's study who were accepted and so encouraged in their pain by others in the dorm, the psalmist's pain is inseparable from social rejection. In the psalmist's case, the pain experience also *causes* social rejection, further exacerbating the pain. The psalmist's condition shares similarities, too, with the experiences of many disabled persons. A disability comes with its own pains, some of which isolate the person from others. Sometimes the isolation is simply a product of being unable to participate in activities; sometimes others actively taunt or shun the one disabled.

From the beginning of Psalm 22, we are drawn into the psalmist's pathos with an anguished cry. But this opening address also hints of hope by demonstrating familiarity and proximity to God, "*My* God, *my* God." Furthermore, as the psalm continues, we read reference to God's earlier help for the psalmist's community and person, as the psalmist looks to and trusts in God's help. Indeed, immediately following the opening cry, we discover a person deeply rooted in a community, a family of generations for whom the psalmist's God has acted in protection and blessing. Remembering earlier help for his ancestors lends hope that the psalmist might experience the same beneficence now. Already in these first verses, the psalmist has situated himself in familial relation to other people.

That the psalmist then describes himself as less than human, reviled and abused by this community, is heartbreaking. His physical distress is described in few, yet evocative, terms. We develop the picture of a person in great and lasting pain, wasting away. This wasting away is not simply physical ("I can count all my bones"). The psalmist is also losing a sense of self, of his intrinsic worth as a human being. Fractured, the psalmist feels less than human ("I am a worm and not a human being"). Furthermore, this feeling is confirmed by the community. He is ostracized ("I am the disdain of people"), taunted ("all who see me make fun of me"), and rejected ("They gape and shake their heads"). The psalmist even fears outright abuse and torture, likening others to terrifying animals who threaten him with attack, so that "I am poured out like water, my heart is like melting wax, . . . my strength is dried up, . . . and my tongue sticks in my jaws." Beyond the psalm's first line, the psalmist does not seem to question God's presence and support; yet that is not enough. Outcast and reviled by others, his condition is unbearable. Other people prove to be necessary to the psalmist's sense of well-being.

This emphasis on the psalmist's social condition is reflected also in the dramatic turn that marks the psalm's second part.[2] The second part clearly follows the first's emphasis on the role of others, but while the psalmist was alienated and reviled in the first part—and partly in relation to God, the psalmist is integrated and celebrated in the second part—in relation to God's community, the body of worshipers among whom the psalmist plays a valuable and positive role. This integration is underscored by its change of audience, from complaint *to* God to declarations *about* God. The psalmist speaks to other people as a member of the community rather than to God about rejection by the community.

The marked shift in the middle of the psalm from complaint to celebration is astonishing. It is especially astonishing that the celebration is embedded in the company of others. In striking contrast to initial complaints of socially exacerbated and isolating pain, the second part of the psalm embeds the psalmist within the community. It is out of his relationship to others that the psalmist then speaks, and his speech reflects a reintegration that is healing. However, this healing applies not only to the psalmist but also to others. The psalmist participates in the community as a person with something unique to offer. His particular experiences situate him to give something special to the community—testimony of living through pain, an embodied witness of personal and social reintegration and value.

Despite the intensity of the psalmist's complaint, finally Psalm 22 is not dominated by it; rather, it is balanced with exclamations of healing reintegration. We witness in Psalm 22 the story of one who knows intense and excruciating pain, compounded by social rejection and loneliness, and who anticipates and articulates a time when his suffering will be cause for celebration insofar as he is reintegrated into the community as a member with the particular contribution of his story.

Campbell's Hero

In his book *The Hero with a Thousand Faces*, Joseph Campbell lays out a theory of personal development influenced and informed especially by world myths and the work of Carl Jung. Considering Psalm 22 in light of Campbell's trajectory of a hero's journey illuminates aspects of the psalm's content and movement and aids our thinking about the experience of pain. Psalm 22 also challenges Campbell's theory in a crucial way; in doing so, the psalm presses us to contemplate the person and role, within his or her social context, of the one who suffers. A brief description of Campbell's archetype of the hero's journey enables us to appreciate how his theory shapes our reading of Psalm 22 to yield new insights into aspects of the experience of pain and possibilities for the person in pain.

Campbell observes that the basic framework for ancient stories of an adventure hero, who can be divine or human, man or woman, is composed of three parts: separation, initiation, and return. At the outset, which may be either voluntary or forced, "[the hero] must put aside his pride, his virtue, beauty, and life, and bow or submit to the absolutely intolerable."[3] Then, the hero faces great trouble punctuated by moments of grace. "Dragons have now to be slain and surprising barriers passed—again, again, and again. Meanwhile there will be a multitude of preliminary victories, unretainable ecstasies, and momentary glimpses of the wonderful land."[4] The process, Campbell concludes, is one of overcoming the ego in order to attain the liberating knowledge of no-self, which he describes as a "godlike" state.[5] "The agony of breaking through personal limitations is the agony of spiritual growth. [. . .] Finally, the mind breaks the bounding sphere of the cosmos to a realization transcending all experiences of form—all symbolizations, all divinities: a realization of the ineluctable void."[6] The hero's return is notable for its characteristic sharing of the "boon," gained from the hero's journey, with other people.

Campbell states that the final realization, which the enlightened hero brings back to others, is good news: "that God is love, that He can be, and is to be, loved, and that all without exception are his children."[7] In the process, there is a reintegration of individuals into the context of such a unifying love. "We are taken from the mother, chewed into fragments and assimilated to the world-annihilating body of the ogre [. . .]; but then, miraculously reborn, we are more than we were. If the God is a [. . .] lord of the universe itself, we then go forth as knowers to whom *all* men are brothers."[8] That Campbell's book has been so popular since its first printing in 1949 attests to the power of this model to understand and interpret common experiences of life trials and to inspire people to find meaning and use out of such difficult times.

Reading Psalm 22 in light of Campbell's theory is indeed illuminating, as I hope to demonstrate below. However, one crucial difference is notable. Campbell appeals to the image of the Bodhisattva for illustration of the hero he has in mind. A Bodhisattva is a kind of god, who upon attaining enlightenment, chooses to return to the world of suffering in order to help other human beings move toward the release of enlightenment. By contrast, the psalmist is in no way divine; rather, he is wholly human. The psalmist has not chosen the experience of pain, but chooses to share his story. It is the psalmist's humanity that makes his

journey and return so powerful. Reading Psalm 22 in light
of Campbell's archetype of the hero's journey, then, invites
reconsideration of what it means to be a hero. The
poignant reality of the psalmist's humanity is paradoxically more meaningful than divinization. In the case of a
pain such as that described and demonstrated in Psalm 22,
the hero is precisely unheroic in his or her normalcy. The
psalmist's "boon," the gift that he brings back to the community, is testimony simply of living with and through
pain as a whole human being. Without the psalmist's full
humanity through the loneliness and agony of pain and as
a reintegrated member of the human community, the story
he tells is impotent. The psalmist is not a larger-than-life
person, more akin to the gods than to mere mortals; he is
no more than, yet completely human. The psalmist's
unheroic heroism embodies his story of lived humanity
and so brings the psalm alive for others. On account of the
psalmist's normalcy, Psalm 22 has power for the very real
people who suffer a pain that hurtles them into a foreign
land with untold terrors, great loneliness, and the imperative challenge of redefining the self.

The psalmist does not meet suffering "head on" with the
intention of using it for some higher purpose. Instead,
thrust into the condition of a great pain that is compounded by alienation from others, the psalmist has no
choice but to address the pain. Its intensity and devastating effects are impossible to ignore. At the psalm's midpoint, everything seems to change. The psalm turns from
complaint and terror marked by loneliness and alienation,
to praise and confidence told among family and friends.
The psalmist even turns his focus to address other people
rather than God. At the psalm's midpoint, where we find a
dramatic shift in perspective and tone, the intention and
import of the text is still grounded in the humanity of its

speaker. And it is out of the psalmist's humanity that we witness an earnest effort to apply his experience of great pain and sorrow to the needs of his community in the context simply of participation and of particular witness to God's interest in and help for the afflicted. Like Campbell's adventure hero who has attained enlightenment, the psalmist by presence and word declares that God is, that God loves, and that there is a fundamental relationship that all people share. Psalm 22 witnesses to perseverance through the agony of pain, the possibility of transformation, and the embodiment of a pained person's intrinsic value as a person and part of the human family.

The author of Psalm 22 moves from a description of and cry out of terrible pain compounded by social rejection to anticipation of relief out of which the psalmist determines to declare hope for others suffering. The psalmist's testimony is not limited, however, only to others who suffer but extends to the entire community. Precisely because of living with and through pain, the psalmist's declaration of God's interest in and dominion over the world and everyone in it is particularly powerful. "Particular" because the psalmist is uniquely marked by his experience. Matt Sanford, founder of Mind-Body Solutions, a yoga studio and non-profit corporation, and author of *Waking: A Passage into Body*, his memoir of paralysis and healing, noted in conversation that it is as though the author of Psalm 22 declares, "See, even I, marked by tragedy and pain, am part of the human family; and precisely because I am so marked, my declaration of God's love and grace is especially powerful."[9] The psalmist thus concludes by finding a use for his pain; and the use matches the pain — from alienation to integration, from social rejection to social contribution.

Inhabiting an Inhuman Country

With the world-shattering cry, "My God, my God, why
have you forsaken me?" the psalmist plunges into a land
of pain. What follows is a kind of journey that the psalmist
undertakes with grief and trembling, following glimpses
of his God, and leaning, when possible, on memories of
substantive strength and support. The psalmist is thrust,
like Campbell's hero, out of what is familiar and into a
lonely land fraught with dangers. The propensity of pain
to make what was familiar and predictable altered and
odd leads many people to liken the experience to inhabiting another world. I cite a few examples here. In the opening chapter of *Illness as Metaphor*, Susan Sontag writes of
the "dual citizenship" that we all hold, "in the kingdom of
the well and in the kingdom of the sick," and "sooner or
later each of us is obliged . . . to identify ourselves as citi-
zens of that other place."[10] Also, Oliver Sacks tells of his
experience losing (and regaining) use of a leg that was "off
the map of the knowable."[11] Kat Duff, who writes of her
experience with chronic fatigue and immune dysfunction
syndrome, concurs, noting, "Illness is a familiar yet foreign landscape existing within the cosmos we inherit and
inhabit as human beings. [. . .] However, [. . . t]here are
very few descriptions of this invisible geography, as if it
were circled by a fog of forgetfulness."[12]

After finding himself thrust into this strange world of
pain, the psalmist orients himself in light of the past experiences of his community. There, the psalmist locates and
recalls the support of God. "In you [our ancestors]
trusted, and they were not embarrassed." Alone and in
trouble, memories of support and help are welcome
glimpses in a landscape whose ground and atmosphere is
pain. Indeed, the psalmist even finds in sarcastic taunts
masquerading as advice, a germ of truth that comforts.

The psalmist's tormentors say, "'Go to God. He will rescue [the psalmist]. He will deliver [the psalmist] because God delights in him.'" The psalmist's response is an introspective memory of God's concern expressed in intimate maternal comfort. "You drew me out from the belly and made me secure on my mother's breast. On you I was cast from the womb. From my mother's belly, you have been my God." On his journey through pain's territory, the psalmist as hero has "momentary glimpses of the wonderful land," such as Joseph Campbell describes.

However, the context is pain. Memories of support and help are welcome but momentary glimpses in the terrifying country of pain, a land permeated by destructive power. The person suffering intractable pain undergoes agonies made terrible both by its effects on the immediate person and by the manner in which it undermines and fractures relationships with other people. Great and chronic pain can wear a person down so much that he or she may feel to be only partly human, his or her personality and general sense of self whittled away along with his or her body. In many cases, the sufferer feels inhuman and others treat him or her differently at best, dismissively or even abusively at worst. For some, their pain has no outward sign. Consequently, the loneliness of pain is compounded by others' disbelief that their professed pain is real, and such disbelief may elicit frustration and anger for the sufferer. For others, their pain is intimately related to visible disability and/or disfigurement. Loneliness is then compounded by the ways in which people consider them—with fascination, pity, dismissal, and even hostility, ways that underscore their difference from others.

Dangers in the land of pain, then, include both the agony of the condition itself and the threat that others' failure to relate wholly to him or her poses to the sufferer's sense of self. Pain thus threatens to undermine a person's humanity. The psalmist's condition and treatment by others lead the psalmist to declare himself outside of the community, even of the human race. "I am a worm and not a man, a joke of a human being and despised by people."[13] Other people's treatment of the psalmist contributes to and confirms his separateness from the "normal" world. "All who see me make fun of me. They gape and shake their heads." In his chapter titled "The Burned," William May writes of the particular difficulties that people face who have suffered severe burns. Frequently disfigured, they may feel repulsive not only to others but also to themselves. Indeed, he writes, "the deepest aversion besets the victim himself. He knows that his very existence now repels others; they recoil first, and only later talk, listen, and venture a smile."[14] Such reactions engender in the burned person feelings of disgust and aversion toward others because their treatment of him or her is different than it is to those who have not suffered such trauma. Feeling alienated by others and actively pushing them away, May observes, "He bears the mark of the uncanny, the German term for which is the *Unheimlich*, literally, the one 'not at home,' the alien, the one driven out beyond the ordinary precincts of hearth and city gates, where no one in his right mind would want to venture, and who therefore sends a shudder through the rest of the community."[15]

Marked by pain that profoundly disfigures the psalmist, whether evident in his body, attitude, and/or behavior, the psalmist's world is changed. The psalmist is alone in a threatening country. The onset of disability effects such a change. To suffer intractable pain is a kind of disability in itself, but it frequently is paired with other kinds, adding injury to the insult, so to speak. The voice of Psalm 22 is the voice of one whose condition is so severe that he feels less than human and in this miserable state is reviled and rejected by others. Exactly what ails the psalmist is not made explicit. Its effects, however, are devastating both to the immediate person ("all my bones are disjointed") and in relation to others ("all who see me make fun of me"). Finally, weak and terrified, the psalmist is undone. "I am poured out like water. [. . .] My heart is like wax, melting in my guts. My strength has dried up like a potsherd, and my tongue sticks in my jaws."

Not only is the psalmist figured as less than human because of his condition, but he in turn also describes those who torment him as non-human. They are likened to wild and threatening beasts—bulls, a lion, and dogs. Wandering through an inhuman landscape, the psalmist asks God to look out for him, for help in his immediate and compromised condition, and for help against the monsters of this land. Pain transforms not only the sufferer but also those people and/or institutions who deal with him or her. In Psalm 22 they are figured as wild beasts, vicious and devouring. Institutions designed to provide care for and/or house the suffering, including insurance and drug companies, hospitals, and nursing homes may themselves become agents of suffering. May notes, "Our total institutions reflect primordial images for sickness and death, images of hiding and devouring prominent in folklore, literature, dream life, and ritual behavior."[16] May cites the proclivity for separation from the world of the sick and aged, as a kind of hiding, and the deleterious financial consequences of treatment as a kind of devouring. He also finds such devouring in action in the deprivation of a patient's identity, especially in chronic cases. The "other" in this part of the sufferer's journey may well become the enemy, a force threatening the sufferer's very life. The psalmist takes an important step in naming these others, in identifying their character and behavior as demeaning, vicious, and rapacious.

Thomas Couser observes that in the genre of pathography, autobiographies of so-called disabled persons are quite new.[17] Also new is the challenge such people are making as a group, a minority marginalized, but not by race, gender, or sexual orientation. Sometimes ignored, treated as less than human, patronized, and even the butt of jokes, these people strive to reclaim their place in society as unique and valuable persons. By naming forces that exacerbate disabilities and insist that the disabled are set apart, such persons declare their place within the dizzingly diverse human family. Identifying aspects of institutions and individual behavior that dehumanize the disabled, challenging these aspects, and demanding change, makes it possible to correct whatever barriers prohibit disabled persons from making contributions to the greater community.

There is a time and place for the one treated as less than human to name antagonistic others as likewise inhuman; and the process paradoxically rehumanizes both. Garret Keizer observes that resisting abuse is an act with positive consequences for the perpetrator as well as the victim. "Because loving him as I love myself, [. . .] I intend to prevent his abuse from destroying us both. In a sense, I am coming to his rescue by refusing to use my own meekness to ensnare him in his own wickednes. [. . .] My prayer for my abuser, like my fight against him, is a refusal to make peace with his damnation."[18] To name as inappropriate and dehumanizing the attitudes of some toward the disabled is to invite honest appreciation of the latter as fully integrated into the human family. A brief guide for the U.S. Dept of Labor Office of Disability Employment

Policy sketches the variety of ways in which people with disabilities encounter "attitudinal barriers," including pity, hero worship, backlash, and denial.[19] Indeed, "Individuals with disabilities are handicapped or disabled by a physical environment that disadvantages them and a culture that excludes or stigmatizes them."[20] Couser notes that among other things, the newly mobilized group of people considered disabled have begun to challenge the notion of disability in the first place. One way is by identifying themselves as differently abled among a society that not only prohibits abilities but also has itself a great many unnamed disabilities. Furthermore, disabled or differently abled, each person is unique, an individual with particular experiences and gifts to offer.

Traversing the lonely landscape of pain and engaging terrifying threats and assaults, a person is transformed. Just before the psalm turns to praise, the psalmist issues a particularly remarkable cry for help from others who compound the psalmist's already fragile condition. It is remarkable for its emphasis on the individual. In addition to asking God to save his *nephesh*, "self," the psalmist iterates "my unique person." Like *nephesh*, this latter word defies a neat one-to-one translation, but it emphasizes the singular nature of the psalmist's person, his particular self, as worthy of deliverance. In its alchemy, pain may act like a refining fire, purifying the person as an individual, clarifying his or her uniqueness. Reflecting on the identity of a person badly burned, May notes that we cannot talk of a new self since the former persists, especially when no brain damage has occurred. Instead, May writes of reclothing the soul.[21] Joseph Campbell describes the process as breaking through the ego to new self-realization. Although the process is a transformation, it is grounded in a persistent self. The alchemist does not add or subtract but refashions out of original elements. Pain transforms; it does not delete or create.

Reflecting on the solitude that pain enforces, Kat Duff writes that while such solitude may add to the distress, it also may serve an important function in the transformation and redefinition of the self. "The isolation and lack of sympathy or understanding that sick people often endure may even be necessary to secure the walls of the container, so that nothing is spilled or shared and the matter inside will reach the point of transmutation. The walled space of illness, like therapy, intensifies the brooding and incubates the egg."[22] In a letter to his brother, Theo, Vincent Van Gogh likens difficult periods in life to the molting time of birds and notes, "One can stay in it [. . .] one can also emerge renewed; but anyhow it must not be done in public [. . .] therefore the only thing is to hide oneself."[23] The psalmist journeys alone through pain, terror, and loss.

Dissolving the Boundaries

The final stage of the hero's journey is return, but it is more than simply coming back. The hero rejoins the community as a changed person. Cast into a foreign land, the psalmist has been crushed in the crucible of pain and denied the company of others, rejected and reviled on account of his condition. Out of that inhuman landscape populated by vicious monsters, the psalmist emerges with something special to share, boon from the journey. The psalmist returns to the community with benefits for the psalmist himself and the greater community as well as for others who suffer. Indeed, an aspect of the psalmist's boon is how sharing it links these three parties inseparably together. The psalmist does not return with a valuable object, but with a story. Telling the story is encouragement to others who suffer, and it is an expression of the psalmist's self-definition as a person of intrinsic value. Furthermore, it benefits the greater community both by demonstrating their supportive acceptance of the one marked by pain and by declaring an enduring goodness that transcends and unites all people. The hero returning from the journey demonstrates "realization of oneness of himself with the world and oneness of the world with its principle of creation. Suffering is integral to this principle, and learning the integrity of suffering is central to the boon."[24]

The psalmist elegantly dissolves barriers between the pained person and others in the context of their shared humanity. The psalmist does not report having been cured, but he is healed. The psalmist tells with a new certainty that God does not reject or deny pain and the one suffering: "God did not disdain or abhor the affliction of the afflicted." Instead, the psalmist declares, sufferer or not, friend or foreigner, all are part of the human family in a shared world of God's making and in God's keeping. "All the ends of the earth," "all the families of the nations," "all the fat of the earth," "all those who go down to the dust," "and whose spirit is not vibrant," are united in the human project of praise. The psalmist's reintroduction, as someone newly defined/refined by great pain and grief, makes a place within the community for others who suffer.

The psalmist's testimony out of pain opens up the possibility that a person's suffering is not a radically isolated event, but is part of a greater whole. Duff writes of a comforting realization that her experience of pain may be participation in something universal. "It feels as though the thin strand of my life is woven back into the web of our world. That may be the answer to my question of how to encompass the painful contradictions and injustices of life."[25] The psalmist's celebration of God's power and help within the greater community extends not only to the psalmist's immediate community but also to all people everywhere ("families of the nations"), even in time to come ("future generations"). Pain is a universal human experience. To tell of it as a person integrated "in the family of things"[26] is to affirm one's connection to all others and simultaneously to affirm the place of others, ground down and alienated by pain, within this family, too.

In the process, the psalmist confidently affirms his humanity and the humanity of others. In contrast to the psalmist's earlier self-description as less than human, and in contrast to descriptions of others as vicious animals, the psalmist rehumanizes both self and others with praise to God in the midst of "my brothers." Indeed, this latter part of the psalm is saturated with references to the humanity of the people among whom the psalmist now situates himself. They include "brothers," "descendants of Israel," "the assembly," "great congregation," "families of the nations," "future generations," "a people yet to be born." Telling his story, the psalmist declares his uniqueness, and does so in the company of others, in the context of sharing ideas and insights out of his particular experience. "The story is one medium through which the communicative body recollects itself as having become what it is, and through the story the body offers itself to others. Recollection of self and self-offering are inseparable, each being possible only as the complement to the other."[27] The psalmist's declaration is a critical part of reclothing his soul, it gives to others who suffer affirmation of their humanity and worth, and it gives to the greater community powerful testimony of enduring goodness and grace.

The psalmist's gift of unifying testimony born of terrific disabling, and/or disfiguring pain is an expression of love.

Sometimes invisible pain is expressed especially psychologically, and its sufferers travel the same roads as those with apparently physical disabilities. Although few people are unfamiliar with the evocative paintings of Vincent Van Gogh, fewer people know that his deepest desire was first to be a parish pastor. In his books, *Van Gogh and God* and *The Shoes of Van Gogh*, Cliff Edwards, religion professor and scholar of Van Gogh's life and work, explores Vincent's faith journey—a journey that led to and is reflected in the paintings for which he is remembered.[28] Faced with social rejection and ostracized from the religious establishment, Vincent became terribly depressed. Unable to practice the ministry he had chosen as pastor to the poor and downtrodden, Vincent turned to art and in doing so, he recrafted his ideas of ministry. In the process, he regained a sense of purpose in life. Vincent made of his art a pulpit from which he preached not doctrine but love, love of the ordinary—nature, creatures, and "the man from the depth of the abyss, *de profundis*—that is the miner" (from Letter 136).[29] Edwards observes, "For Vincent, [. . .] both 'God' and 'love' locate themselves [. . .] in the simplicity of life."[30] This love, Campbell writes, marks the hero who returns.

The psalmist's boon is not shared only with other sufferers, but with the whole congregation, and it extends to all peoples. Well members of the community experience healing through the testimony of the hero who has journeyed through the land of pain as much as those who are in pain. The psalmist, our adventure hero, takes up a song of praise and declares the goodness and purposefulness of the world in a manner that backgrounds pain and foregrounds relationships to others. Margaret Mohrmann writes of her experience as a pediatrician that "the ones we serve" also serve us. Turning around interpretations of the command to love one's neighbor and of the parable of the Good Samaritan who helped the wounded enemy, Mohrmann writes, "my neighbor is the Samaritan, my neighbor is the one who shows me mercy. I am not the Samaritan; I am the one who needs the Samaritan."[31] The consequences of this up-side-down perspective are profound. Among those who find healing in the psalmist's return and testimony are the ones who seemed well all along. Declaration within the human family of God's sovereignty and praiseworthiness by one such as this psalmist is compelling testimony. On account of the psalmist's pain, his terrifying and lonely experience, the psalmist's posture of wonder and awe are particularly powerful.

The psalmist demonstrates that pain does not have the final word, that the psalmist's harrowing journey through pain was not the final chapter of his life. The psalmist attains special knowledge on account of his suffering, new awareness of connections, and appreciation of the existence of goodness and help. The terrible journey through pain is an aspect of his life experience that situates the psalmist with something to share. The psalmist did not choose his pain or graciously accept suffering with the idea of using it for some greater purpose in an act of superhuman or martyring heroism. The psalmist speaks as an ordinary human being. His heroism is simply living through pain as a productive part of the whole community. Duff writes of the wisdoms that she has learned in illness—countless things that the well pass by, take for granted, or lose. She concludes, "I hope I do not forget when I get well."[32] The heroism of the psalmist does not elicit worship but simply attention.

8

Moving Pain out of the Center (Psalm 6)

◁▷

*"My eye darkens with vexation, worn out by all
these who hold me back."*

To stand up and takes one's place within the greater community and there declare that help is knit into the fabric of
the world and that participation does not require perfect
health and happiness is to bring treasure back from pain
with a special knowledge, which those who have suffered
greatly can offer. In the previous chapter, we saw how the
author of Psalm 22 takes such a stance. The author of
Psalm 6 takes a different stance, one of rejection and
denunciation. In Psalm 6, we witness the determined
rejection of forces that diminish a person, that hold him or
her back from growth and development despite conditions of pain. To take a stand of protest against such forces
requires not only great courage but also assuming control
of one's life and experience. It is to claim one's experiences
for oneself, not simply as the product of outside agency
that victimizes into inaction.

Taking control of the experience of pain is paradoxically
inseparable in Psalm 6 from moving the pain out of the
center of the psalmist's life. This is partly demonstrated by
the manner in which initial questions about God's part in

causing the psalmist's pain are left unresolved. Determining God's role in the psalmist's pain changes from questions of agency to certainty of support. Taking control of the experience of pain includes accepting irresolution of questions about meaning and focusing instead on how to live fully despite the pain. We find in Psalm 6 a three-part process: first a focus on the pain itself and pleading for a cure, then cessation of all activity except grief, and finally a strident call of protest that concludes in a triumphant tone of vindication and hope.

Psalm 6 shares characteristics with the other psalms that we have considered. Among these characteristics are its association of the psalmist's painful condition with the punitive anger of God; the whole-person experience of pain; the sense that after death, all relationship to God is severed; and the identification of enemy-others who contribute either immediately or indirectly to the psalmist's pain. Despite such shared elements, Psalm 6 as a whole gives us occasion to consider them in the context of something more — a shift of focus and power that moves pain out of the center of the psalmist's attention in defiance of what holds her back. After the probing questions of why and pleas for help, and after grief over the losses that intractable pain exacts, we hear a new determination to reject whatever compromises the integrity and strength of the one in pain. Taking control of her experience, the psalmist concludes with confidence and hope — confidence in support and hope in the ultimate defeat of whatever conspires to diminish a person.

Changing styles of speech, from complaint to grief to denunciation of what causes pain, mark Psalm 6's shift in focus. There is change not only *between* these three general movements, but also *within* them, demonstrated by the psalmist's thinking and behavior. Within the context of complaint, addressed to God, we witness a change from thinking of God's punitive anger as a reason for pain to thinking of God as an interested and caring healer, a companion in pain, and one whose relationship with the psalmist may be reason enough for God to save her from death. Within the context of grief, addressed as much introspectively as to anyone else, readers witness movement from the psalmist's lament of exhaustion and wasting away to candid identification of the problem. At this point, the psalmist's focus moves from self to others, as the psalmist recognizes her feelings of "vexation," and then identifies those who prohibit the psalmist's full expression and development as the cause of such feelings. Within the context of denunciation, the psalmist moves from identification and rejection of "troublemakers" to confidence that the psalmist is strongly supported and finally to a triumphant expression of hope that the tables will turn and malevolent forces will turn away shaking and in shame.

In the process of the psalm, the psalmist goes from feeling the victim of a terrible agency outside of her control, to self-reflection that allows a period of grief and self-pity, to active denunciation and rejection of whatever may worsen her condition. This last is coupled with a sense of confidence and hope. However, the confidence and hope are not articulated in terms of relief from pain; rather, they concern anticipation of triumph over those forces that exacerbate the psalmist's distress by prohibiting her own expression of agency and power. In other words, if the pain is finally assuaged, we can only guess at it and attribute it to the psalmist's new attitude and focus. The identification of "those who hold me back" and the denunciation of troublemakers demonstrates renewed vigor and determination to live as well and as fully as possible, which may mean doing so in the face of pain.

With this conclusion, Psalm 6 leaves unanswered the questions raised at its beginning about the genesis and purpose of pain. Changing its focus without resolution of issues introduced at the beginning, the psalm invites readers to consider how thinking differently about pain may actually relieve its most vicious expression. Author of *Safe at Last in the Middle Years, Aged by Culture and Declining to Decline*, Margaret Morganroth Gullette writes of an early injury's pain and its relationship to an arthritis that she now associates simply with aging.[1] In telling her story, Gullette relates the manner in which she initially thought about her pain, the problems raised by the first physician that she consulted, her contemplation of suicide, and the manner in which she changed her thinking (again) about the causes and effects of her pain. She concludes her essay by noting that she has finally determined that the pain of her arthritis is simply an "ordinary pain," and it is not all there is of/to her.[2] As such, it merits no drama, "no rapid response," but rather an effort to live out of the interests and abilities that she has. By moving pain out of the center of her attention and life, she has rendered it much less terrifying and destructive.

Shifting one's thinking about pain is seldom as neatly linear a process as we find in Psalm 6. Nevertheless, for people like Gullette, it allows a reintegration of the self that accounts for the continued reality of pain simply as part of a many-sided life full of possibility and promise. Disallowing pain to continue to fracture and paralyze such a life means identifying the pain for what it is and determining to focus on what one is nevertheless able and wanting to do and be. Frequently, such a shift in focus away from one's pain actually works to mitigate it. Simple distraction is one example. Another is refiguring treatment. Susan Greenhalgh tells of her experiences of chronic pain and how abuses in medical practice contributed to her degeneration physically, mentally, and socially. When she determined to reject the patronizing and controlling method of her physician, her health improved dramatically. This particular physician, whom Greenhalgh calls Dr. D., failed to listen to Greenhalgh, instead superimposing problems on her and proceeding to treat these false problems, grossly exacerbating her pain. Greenhalgh's story relates a particularly egregious case of disenfranchising a person in pain so that all control is abdicated and the physician's story of her pain takes precedent over any other.[3]

John Sarno pointedly warns against physicians taking such an approach, arguing that it does much more harm than good. His theory of Tension Myositis Syndrome (TMS) locates the problem of back pain in psychological processes, which cause a physiological reaction that starves muscles of blood. Sarno champions a person's ability to gain control over his or her own pain by noting how anxieties and fears contribute to or even cause the pain. Sarno reveals as misleading "structural" diagnoses, such as a herniated disc or "pinched nerve," for chronic pain in the back, neck, shoulders, buttocks, and legs. Such "conventional diagnoses unwittingly contribute to the severity and persistence of back pain because they frighten and intimidate."[4] Encouraging people to consider how their back pain masks psychological and emotional pains, Sarno effectively directs people to move their pain out of the center, and in the process, he notes that most find relief. Rather than prescribing expensive treatments, Sarno observes, "The best medicine: releasing the potential within individuals to heal themselves."[5]

In its expression and interpretation of the psalmist's pain, the psalm moves from God to self to others in a tone of increasing self-respect and control of circumstances. The psalmist moves from fear of punishment and a sense of helplessness, with God as the addressee, to poignant complaint and grief over her individual condition, to criticism of others for contributing to the psalmist's pain, and finally to confidence in vindication. Pain is not abolished, but it moves out from the center of the psalmist's attention, and in that process, the pain is mitigated. One facet of this change is evident in the manner in which questions about meaning, fore-grounded at the beginning of the psalm, are left unresolved as the focus turns instead to the practical problem of managing the effects of pain. Exploring this matter is the subject of the first section below. Following the psalm's development, I then discuss the nature and implications of the psalm's central expression of grief. In the concluding section, I note how the psalmist assumes control and determines to reject whatever interferes with her health and development.

"Holding Fragments"[6]

Beliefs about order, purpose, goodness, and evil tend to crowd to the front when a person is confronted with chronic pain. If the sufferer is a person of monotheistic faith or is informed by such a cultural context, these beliefs may be bound up in how he or she understands God and God's role in the world. The psalmist begins by reflecting certain ideas about God and suffering, ideas that suffering is not purposeless but comes from God, and that it comes from God for certain reasons. "Do not discipline me in your anger. Do not chasten me in your rage." This exclamation supposes ideas about God as a passionate judge—punishing out of righteous anger, inflicting pain in order to correct and instruct. However, the psalm also undermines these early ideas in several ways. It lacks reference to the psalmist's wrongdoing, it includes no expression of penitence, and it proffers alternative images of God as a gracious healer. Furthermore, the structure of Psalm 6 sets the introductory exclamation apart from the rest of the psalm, leaving the matter unresolved.

The literary context of Psalm 6 underscores ambivalence about the role of God in the experience of pain and demonstrates aspects of the psalmist's cultural context that consequently shape her experience of pain. Although the book of Psalms was not composed as a unit, at one time and in the order that it has come to us, the psalms preceding Psalm 6 provide a window into the psalmist's cultural context insofar as they relate some of the ideas and images that are prominently represented within the Old Testament/Hebrew Bible. Furthermore, given the final editorial shape of the Psalter as it has come down to us, the psalms that precede Psalm 6 form a literary context that shapes readers' ideas about Psalm 6. Knowing something about these preceding psalms, then, aids our understanding of Psalm 6.

Psalms 1 and 2 are not only the first psalms but also reflect two legs on which the whole book (arguably "the whole Book") stands — Torah and monarchy. Psalm 1 emphasizes the importance of God's instruction (Torah) and the delight that knowing and living by that instruction gives a person. Psalm 2 emphasizes the importance of God's relationship and agreement with the people as a defined group, a nation, led by a king understood to be God's beloved, chosen regent. Given their prominence throughout the Hebrew Bible, these themes are fundamental to the psalmist's cultural and ideological context and so provide critical pieces in the puzzle of how she understands and assimilates her experience of pain.

With Psalms 3 and 4 we hear voices of concern related to the fear and distress that Psalm 6 tells. Psalm 3, introduced as "A Psalm of David, when he fled from his son Absalom," develops an idea from Psalm 2—God's protection and support for the king. In Psalm 3, the speaker begins with an exclamation of fear and/or intimidation in the face of strong enemies but moves quickly to expression of confidence in God's support. Psalm 4 takes up again the sense of fear and distress, but makes the experience and the subsequent expression of confidence in God's help more democratic than Psalm 3. That is, in Psalm 4, the speaker could be anyone and provides advice to anyone. Both Psalms 3 and 4 refer to lying down and sleeping in the safety of God. While Psalm 5 begins with distress familiar to us from Psalms 3 and 4, the complaint is more sustained; and instead of reference to lying down and sleeping in safety, 5:2-3 tells of crying in the morning to God. All of these psalms warn against wickedness and express assurance that those who maintain righteousness will be protected and made secure by God, in contrast to wrongdoers, who should expect divine rejection and punishment.

In such a context, Psalm 6 is a striking development. The speaker begins by expressing concern that she will be or is the object of God's corrective punishment, so far conforming to preceding ideas of pain as the byproduct of God's discipline. However, the speaker's sin is not clarified or even identified. Rather, the focus is on the speaker's condition itself, which is described as an overwhelming disquiet that has affected the psalmist's whole person. Exactly what injury or illness is at the root of this general distress is not clear; we know only that it causes groaning and much crying. This is a condition that the preceding psalms identify with punishment for the wicked (and note that the psalmist pleads for help first in terms of being spared God's wrath). That the psalmist does not confess to having sinned leads the reader to suspect that although the psalmist's suffering may look like God's punishing judgment, it is not, or it is undeserved.[7]

Indeed, there is no reasoning or description that attends the negative command that introduces the psalm. We read simply, "do not discipline me in your wrath, do not chasten me in your rage." That these are the first words of the psalm, lends a sense of urgency, even emergency. It is as though the psalm begins in the middle; as though we have entered late into the room of a conversation well on its way. Its next exclamation mirrors this sense of crisis, but with a different, more conciliatory, even pleading tone: "Be gracious to me, O God, for I am feeble; heal me, God, for my bones are shaking." Together, these verses tell two sides of the psalmist's hope, and in doing so, they tell two sides of the psalmist's theology—do not discipline or chasten (both verbs suggest deserved punishment enacted in order to teach a lesson), rather be gracious and heal (conditions in which punishment is moot).

With the psalmist's prayer, we find not only the expression of desire for relief but also the bases of a theodicy that wrestles with the relationship of ideas of a God who is all-powerful and just, but also gracious and merciful. The psalmist reveals assumptions about God both as judge, who may punish with a righteous anger that is painful and instructive, and as gracious—demonstrating special favor, an attribute that the psalmist associates here with healing. There is profound ambivalence in these assumptions. The ambivalence is sustained also in verses 3-4 where we read the intensity and effects of the psalmist's pain in the context of paradoxical ideas about God. The stuttered "and you, YHWH—how long?" underscores the magnitude of the psalmist's pain. It does not make sense as a full sentence, but is rather the lurching expression of someone overcome and grasping for help. Complaining that her whole self shakes, the psalmist looks to God as the one responsible, if not for the pain, then at least for determining the duration of suffering—"how long?"[8] Yet the psalmist juxtaposes this association of God's judgment with suffering to God's compassion as expressed in the relief of pain. The psalmist lays side-by-side paradoxical assumptions about God's character—that God is judgmentally responsible for suffering, yet also mercifully compassionate.

The project of theodicy recognizes and attempts to deal with such a challenge of understanding the existence of pain and suffering in a world created by a loving and all-powerful God. Theorizing about pain makes it possible to observe dispassionately the ambivalence of such assumptions and move on. Really facing pain brings such paradox into sharp and troubling relief. It is one thing, and a valuable thing, to debate the variety of ways one might reconcile ideas of God with the reality of pain; but it is quite another thing to face such pain—one's own or another's, and come up with a response that is sensible and appropriate. The first group of articles in the book *Pain Seeking Understanding* considers the distinction between theoretical and practical theodicy in a manner that accounts for voices such as the one we hear in Psalm 6. Larry Bouchard writes in the book, "Practical theodicy will authorize the afflicted to call God into account and yet also attend to the promise of God's solidarity with the afflicted."[9] This is the only theodicy that can make sense of the psalmist's ambivalence between a God who both causes pain for punitive instruction and is a gracious healer and companion in the suffering. It succeeds less by making sense than by allowing a place for irreconcilable ways of thinking about God's part in the experience of pain. Psalm 6 demands such a practical theodicy as it juxtaposes paradoxical elements. "Juxtaposition," Bouchard writes, "is an alternative to positing a total framework of thought."[10]

Just as Bouchard follows his explanation of justification with the comment, "I do mean to leave incomplete the bridges of thought between the stories, images, or actions we juxtapose,"[11] reconciling opposing attributes of God is not finally what occupies the psalmist's attention and energy. They are left, unresolved, as "incomplete bridges of thought." Margaret Mohrmann observes, "[Theodicy] is less the abstract reconciliation of propositions about God, more the work of making things of form and beauty out of lived anxiety and pain."[12] What finally occupies the psalmist is standing up for herself against forces that would compromise her ability to grow and develop. It is these malevolent forces that the psalmist addresses with a strong denunciation, and she confidently asserts that God supports her rejection of "troublemakers" and "all those who hold me back." The psalmist does not immediately shift, however, from complaint and questions of meaning to assuming control with a positive determination; rather, first she grieves. In the center of the poem we find the psalmist deep in sadness, mourning the losses that pain has exacted.

The Fulcrum of Grief

Psalm 6 never clearly identifies the reason for the psalmist's distress. Even references to God's anger are not anchored in notice of what the psalmist may have done to elicit such anger—some misbehavior or fault, or for raising the problem of his or her condition.[13] What is clear is the intensity of suffering. The structure of the psalm underscores these impressions—irresolution about the genesis and purpose of the psalmist's pain, and its severity as something both devastating and demanding address. As it develops, the psalm leads readers away from attempts to reconcile ideas about God's character, purpose, and role toward simply acknowledging the pain, with its attendant issues and problems.

With verse 6, the psalmist ceases crying to, complaining, and bargaining with God, and instead turns her attention inward. "I am weary with my moaning." It is an exclamation with no clear addressee. Sodden with resignation, it emerges from the psalmist's core and goes out both to no one and to everyone. In Psalm 6, we have only the poet's words, a simple, spare commentary on extraordinary grief. "I am weary with my moaning, every night I soak my sleeping place with tears and dissolve my sick-bed." The grief is an end in itself. In this verse we hear exhausted mourning over the losses of previous abilities and future plans or goals that pain effects. Such grief reflects the fact that a person dealing with chronic pain is changed, and the previous pain-free self is no more.

Pain imposes a change that includes loss. The loss of a previous pain-free self frequently means the loss of much of what may have defined a person's sense of who and how he or she is. Bringing her experience as a pediatrician and theological ethicist to bear on instruction and practice at the University of Virginia, Margaret Mohrmann explains, "whatever else is going on and however else they seek to make sense of and deal with this terrible experience, it is important that people in pain acknowledge that they will be changed."[15] As pain wrecks its havoc, that it changes a person becomes undeniable. When Kat Duff came down with chronic fatigue and immune dysfunction syndrome (CFIDS), she says, "[the effects] unraveled my life and sense of myself in a matter of months."[16] The sense expressed in the center of Psalm 6 is of hitting the bottom and turning inward to grieve. The only thing the psalmist does or even can do, is cry. Verse 6 is the nadir of the psalm.

However, verse 6 is not the end; grief does not have the final word. Instead, this verse is a kind of fulcrum on which the psalm tilts. Hope is built into the structure of the psalm. The fullness of mourning makes novelty possible. Recognizing that one's pain is chronic and intractable means recognizing that one's life is different on account of pain's presence in it. Gullette writes that everybody knows that when you are in pain, you do anything to minimize it, but "What no one ever talks about convincingly, [. . .] is how your identity tries to change when your body changes."[17] Out of great grief comes growing awareness of the necessity to craft a new self out of the old, a new self that accounts for both the intimate presence of pain and the vitality of the one suffering. Susan Greenhalgh also struggled with increasing pain and decreasing options under the domineering and manipulative care of her physician until, like Gullette, she contemplated taking her own life. Instead, she adopted a new way of being. The company and counsel of friends and family, and the opinion of a second physician, encouraged her to recraft her self with empowering feminist principles to be less the "good girl," silently complying and eager to please, and more authentically true to herself.

Years of medical practice, research, and simple observation have led Sarno to conclude that most chronic back pain (including pain in the shoulders, neck, buttocks, and legs) is the combined result of a person's tension (frequently associated with a drive to excel in work and relationships) and physicians' "structural" diagnoses of injury and physiological deterioration. The beginning of relief from pain, Sarno observes, is as simple as "confronting the fact that tension can produce back pain."[18] Considering the "pain in *emotional terms*, [. . .] the tension will ease to produce a *physical reaction*" of relief.[19] Such a shift requires that a person adopt a whole new way not only of thinking about her pain but also of being, in general. Gaining control over one's life is frequently coupled with gaining control over one's pain.

The psalmist's perspective, attitude, and behavior begin to change out of the depths of grief, and they do so in ways that echo and alter her previous manner. The psalm moves from verse 6 to verses that pair with preceding ones.[20] Changes in the psalmist's focus and address underlie this movement. In the first part, God is the addressee and pain is the focus as the psalmist cries out to God for relief; in the last part of the psalm, the author takes charge in addressing others, and the focus is on relief from malevolent troublemakers. Following the matched pairs around verse 6, we see that verses 5 and 7 tell of wasting away/nearing death, and the others party to this are respectively "you, YHWH" and "all those who hold me back." Verses 4 and 8 both express the action of turning, but they do so with different verbs and subjects. In verse 4, the verb is *shuv*, ("returning") and its subject is God; in verse 8, the verb is *sur* ("turning away") and its subject is troublemakers. The request for help in verse 4, for drawing out the psalmist's life and delivering her on account of God's kindness, is answered in verse 8 by God's attention and the troublemakers' desisting. The terrifying condition and desperate question "how long?!" in verse 3 is answered by verse 9: God has heard and accepted. The psalmist's weakness and disquiet in verse 2 (and 3a) are mirrored by the enemies' shame and disquiet in verse 10.

This leaves the first verse standing alone, leaving unresolved the question of whether or not God's punishing wrath has anything to do with the psalmist's present distress. Independent from the others, these two verses (1 and 6) become a kind of pair that situates the last part of the psalm. Indeed, the exclamation in verse 1, with its attendant question(s) stands unanswered by any other verse; and the psalmist's pain, most poignantly demonstrated by verse 6 is unassuaged. From the psalm's midpoint to its end, the focus is external to the psalmist and God's part is described (in the third person), not shown (in the second or first person). The psalmist turns away from addressing God and away from introspective grief to address, with caustic criticism, the ones who make trouble, also identified as the ones who hold the psalmist back.

Gullette considered taking her own life after visiting an orthopedist who told her to expect a steady and painful decline in her general health and physical ability, and the doctor did so in the context of ideas about Gullette's personal responsibility and fault. "He implied that I had had control over my back—my pain, my life—that I had regularly abused."[21] The pain and her prognosis elicited great "grief over my lost future."[22] Gulette then consciously determined to reject his association of her condition with dismissive blame and patronizing authority and, remarkably, the back pain subsided as the troublesome disk was reabsorbed by her body. Now, she lives with the intermittent pain of arthritis, a pain that she associates simply with aging. Pain no longer dominates her thoughts with fear and anxiety over what the pain might "mean" and how it might progress. Gullette has moved pain out from the center of her life and has found it to be manageably reduced. Acknowledging the loss of a pain-free self and simply recognizing the reality of pain in one's life may bring its own relief. Marni Jackson writes, "As soon as I give in and accept that Pain isn't going to leave, I instantly begin to feel better. Less cornered. I take a deep breath . . ., and at last I fall asleep."[23]

Denouncing Limits

No matter the condition, to be fully alive is to be present to real circumstances and to determine one's way, as an integrated person, within those circumstances. Like Jackson, finding a relieving freedom may mean simply acknowledging the persistent nature of one's pain. For others, it may require more actively denouncing other things or people who keep one back from reaching out for ways to grow and develop in the midst of pain. For yet others, it may be that the prohibitions of others or of society in general are finally at the root of the pain itself and as such must be identified and managed accordingly. In all cases, the pained person takes initiative and control to move pain out of the center of his or her life in order to get on with the matter of being whole and alive even in the face of continuing pain.

Unclear about the genesis and purpose of her pain, and "holding fragments" of ideas about God's agency and help in the context of continuing pain, the psalmist grieves; but out of grief, the psalmist expresses a new thing—annoyance and criticism of "those who hold me back." Indeed, verse 7 continues in the tone of introspection and private grief, but at the end of the sentence, the psalmist identifies the trouble—"those who hold me back." After tears, the psalmist seems to set her feet firmly beneath her and identifies a problem external to her. The psalmist moves away from looking to God to cure the pain, and focuses instead on confronting those whom the psalmist identifies as compromising her growth and development. The two Hebrew phrases that identify these malevolent others leave open the possibility of understanding them as non-human forces. Instead of identifying them specifically as other people, the psalmist describes them by their effects — "those who restrict me" and "those who make trouble/sorrow."[24] And the psalmist declares that she is *vexed* by them.

Such annoyance or anger in this context reflects a healthy sense of identity and self-worth. In some cases, anger can be toxic and destructive to the one angry and to any or all nearby. Recent studies have shown that anger can actually contribute to higher blood pressure and increased risk of heart attack and stroke.[25] However, expressing anger in a direct and controlled manner may relieve such risks, and in any case, reflects a sense of self-respect.[26] Garret Keizer confesses that he is "unable to commit to any messiah who doesn't knock over tables."[27] He concludes his book by noting, "The belief behind everything I have said is that anger can be controlled without being destroyed, and expressed without necessarily leading to destruction."[28] As an antidote to behavior that belittles or compromises a person, vexation such as that expressed by the psalmist is not only healthy and enabling but has a respectable place within the "emotional repertoire of any evolved human being," including one who is deeply religious.[29]

The psalmist denounces those who make trouble, demands that they go away, and then expresses confidence that they will do so, shaking and ashamed. The psalm moves from fear to confidence, from anxiety to agency, all within the context of illness. It is not clear that the psalmist has been relieved of her suffering at the end of the psalm, but she is confident that God has heard, and "accepted [the] prayer." The psalmist reinterprets her experience and suggests that pain and illness need not preclude confidence that God hears and "accepts prayer." Rather than following such expression of confidence with a description of relief from pain, the psalmist reports taking charge of her condition, rejecting those who would do her ill. "Minimally, a practical theodicy understands suffering and evil by resisting the effects of the consequences of suffering and evil."[30] There is no explicit notice that the psalmist's physical situation has changed by the end of the psalm, but her attitude and focus have. Psalm 6 tells of gaining control over one's life, of speaking out against whoever or whatever interferes with the psalmist's personal development.

In her book *Suffering*, Christian theologian Dorothee Soelle writes of three stages of suffering, each a process of change involving speech, relationships, and power.[31] Soelle's theory provides insight into the manner in which Psalm 6 moves from complaint to grief to denunciation. In the first stage, Soelle explains that the sufferer cannot speak and feels alone and powerless. While the poet of Psalm 6 is not mute and her address to God presumes some kind of relationship, the manner of speech and relationship at the psalm's beginning connotes distance from other people and a distinct sense of powerlessness. The second stage of suffering, which Soelle calls "the stage of lament, of articulation, the stage of the psalms," she describes as one of lamenting speech, communication, and acceptance and conquest in existing structures. Psalm 6 is indeed a psalm of lament in which the psalmist describes her pain and articulates its implications for herself and for her relationship to God and others. That the psalmist does not tell of relief as an immediate response to the psalmist's prayer but instead becomes "introverted" in verse 6 suggests a kind of (weary) acceptance of the psalmist's condition. Identifying psalmic literature with the second stage of suffering, Soelle does not describe how the psalms may also express the further transformation to overcome powerlessness within the context of "changed structures" that is characteristic of her theory's third stage.[32] Yet the author of Psalm 6 continues to change and develop after grief, expressing new conditions of self-respect, a sense of power on account of God's attention, and a reversal of fates whereby those who caused the psalmist trouble and distress are themselves disquieted and shamed.

Despite the psalm's beginning, with its attention to pain and the anxiety such pain provokes, its resolution does not articulate the absence of pain. Rather, pain simply is no longer the psalmist's focus. Through a development associated with relationships — to God, self, and others — the psalmist gains a tone of self-respect, confidence, and hope. Indeed, the psalmist seems to suggest first that the source of pain is important, though it may be difficult to identify, but finally that it does not matter. "It is not the intellectual history of the question [of theodicy] that impinges, but its immediate power to shape the sufferer's experience of the divine in her life and to frame her capacity to meet the present crisis."[33] The psalmist's pain and matters of theodicy become secondary to denouncing whatever prohibits her and recognizing God's support in rejecting them. The psalmist moves pain out from the center of her attention, and in the process, she finds relief.

9

Meanwhile the World Goes On
(Psalm 102)

✎

*"My days are like a spreading shadow, and I dry up
like vegetation. But you YHWH dwell forever."*

Any discussion of pain is incomplete without accounting
for the inescapable, radically common fact of death. We
have already seen, expressed in other psalms, the resistance to death that is natural in life. Yet, as Wendell Berry
observes, "any definition of health that is not silly must
include death."[1] Psalm 102 gives us occasion to reflect on
aspects of aging and the inevitable reality of death in a
manner that is eminently healthy. It does not romanticize,
whitewash, or otherwise dismiss the pain of degeneration
and loneliness that frequently accompany the dying
process. In the style of candor and honesty about the
human condition that characterizes the psalms and
endears them to us, Psalm 102 poignantly tells the troubles of a dying person. However, in keeping with the
dynamic character of the psalms, the psalmist's thinking
about his condition changes, increasing in scope from an
individual's suffering to the greater world and the God
who created and sustains it. In the process, readers hear a
relieving transition from the stranglehold of pain to an
opening appreciation of a wide world that will continue

long after the psalmist's death. Attending this transition is wonder at a limitless God who deigns to be intimately involved even in the limitations of life.

Any person's pain is a function of his or her finitude, a finitude inseparable from its implications of imperfection. A poem that continues to ring for me with a musical meaning, even years after I first read it, is Mary Oliver's "Wild Geese." The rhythm of the poem underscores the meaning of its spare words, a meaning that neatly shifts, twice, to result in a whole that embraces the paradoxes of human finitude. I note Oliver's poem here because the sense of it is in keeping with some of what makes Psalm 102 powerfully relevant to our inquiry about pain. I am reluctant to tell what a poem is "about," yet I find something at the heart of Oliver's "Wild Geese" that is also at the heart of Psalm 102. These poems, one modern and one ancient, tell in distinct voices the imperfection of human beings, our inability to "get it all just right" in the context of our finitude.[2]

"Wild Geese" begins by addressing the reader with an expression of comforting acceptance, despite personal imperfections, and grants permission to the body to "love what it loves." Then, in intimate solidarity, the poet acknowledges the particular yet common experience of despair. The poem shifts with the first "meanwhile" to remind, "the world goes on," and then it turns panoramic to take readers, with "the clear pebbles of the rain," over vast and varied landscapes. When the poem shifts again, it does so with our eyes on the wild geese "flying home" and declaring that each individual has a place within the greater family of the world.

Oliver's "meanwhile," in the middle of the poem, elegantly brings together the frailty and imperfections of any given human life with the awesome nature of the world of which each person finally is a part, seemingly insignificant, but a part nonetheless, with a place of intrinsic value. Although pain can dominate a person's world, it is dwarfed by the immensity of a universe filled with beauty and all kinds of life. Pain, especially the pain that clings close to death, brings together the paradoxical experiences of oneself both as unique and individually important, and as only a tiny part of the world that preceded, will succeed, and is at any moment much greater than any one life.

Psalm 102 grapples with such pain, lamenting the frailty and failing of a body nearing its end, of a person who once enjoyed a place of standing but now feels cast aside — sleepless and alone, with no desire to eat or hope for recovering. In Psalm 102, we hear complaints of chronic pain in the context of a life of numbered days. Frequent references to the psalmist's mortality, such as notice of "my days" passing away in comparison with the eternalness of God, suggest such an understanding. Although some other psalms that we have considered expressed a sense of being close to death, they make sense in the context of a life of indefinite duration; Psalm 102 is the voice of a person dying.[3]

In this condition, the psalmist focuses first on the pain that attends his road to death and laments this pain with heart-rending references to present loneliness and former strengths withered away. Echoing a similar sentiment, Garrison Keillor laments, "One day you're young and brilliant and sullen to your elders, and the next you're getting junk mail from the American Association of Retired Persons and people your very own age are talking about pension plans and the prostate."[4] As the psalm progresses, the author's thinking turns to the wide world and to the infinite nature of God. In the process, the psalmist acknowledges the breadth and depth of the world and its people in a manner that disallows preoccupation with any one individual. Keillor notes, "A sense of mortality should make us smarter [. . .] You plant trees. You cook spaghetti sauce. You talk to children."[5] In what follows, I explore first how the matter of human finitude and its relationship to theodicy finds voice in Psalm 102, and then what the implications of such finitude are in the context of the pain of the dying. Finally, I ask how the psalmist's tone situates his dying and what implications this has for the relationship between what is finite and what is infinite, between human beings and God.

Little Less than Angels

Considering the wonder of the world—earth and heavens, starry skies and newborn babies, another psalmist (that of Psalm 8) asks God, in gratitude and awe, "In the scope of this world's great wonder, what is a human being that you should pay such attention to him or her? Yet you have made human beings little less than gods, crowned us with glory and majesty, and given us control over the whole world." Indeed, we enjoy great privilege and power in and over the world and its inhabitants. That observation, in the context of a faith that declares God to be the creator and sustainer of this wonderful world and that believes God specially loves people as individuals, leads at some point to the question of pain. Given the power, justice, and love of God, why should people suffer debilitating pain?

This is the central question of theodicy. Attempting to make sense out of this problem, people frequently concentrate on defining what or who God is. The results vary. Some claim that God's power really is limited, though some add that God chose to limit God's own power in order to allow for human freedom. Such arguments are often made in order to champion human freedom. God limited God's power in order to allow people full freedom. Other people, observing that we cannot know the meaning and end of all events, argue that God ultimately works in all of our experiences of pain to our benefit. Suffering either teaches us something or keeps us from getting involved in another, even worse situation. We simply do not know it at the time. Consequently, the reasoning goes, we should accept on faith that God allows us present suffering in order to effect something better. Yet another way to manage the problems of theodicy is to argue that God does not will or cause pain but is with us in our pain.

Such attempts to reconcile the existence of pain with the existence of a loving and powerful God are frequently well developed and reasonable within the constraints of philosophical inquiry and/or faith. Finally, however, although there is something compelling about each one, none of these arguments is entirely satisfactory. In their determination to figure out what and who God is, they fail to appreciate the importance of asking what and who people are.[6] Attempting to define, understand, and interpret God's ways is much more difficult than inquiring first into the manner and ways of human beings. Such asking about the nature of what it means to be human is to acknowledge the wonder both that we are little less than angels and that we are dust. It is to wrestle, with the poet of Psalm 102, with terrible pain, loneliness, and the anxiety of our mortality while appreciating that generations come and go, the world is wide and wonderful, and God goes on forever.

To be human is to be a creature, made of the stuff of earth. Such materialness comes with limits, the most obvious being that of our mortality. To be human is also to have and to exercise freedom, the freedom to make

choices about our lives from the smallest, most insignificant details to the greatest decisions. Such freedom means
that we make mistakes and some of those mistakes cause
pain—our own and to others. Daniel Sulmasy, trained as
both a medical doctor and bioethicist, is a Franciscan friar
who teaches at New York Medical College. His contribution to the articles concerning theodicy and the practice of
medicine, edited by Margaret Mohrmann and Mark
Hanson, focuses first on this matter of what humans are in
order to consider the problem of theodicy. He concludes
that human beings are creatures, materially constituted,
having consciousness, are essentially free, bear intrinsic
dignity, and are finite. Sulmasy associates dignity with the
"inalienable meaning or value" that comes simply from
being human. Although he does not articulate it as such, I
add that dignity is directly related to the exercise of our
consciousness and freedom in the context of creaturely
materialness. The responsibility that comes with the freedom to choose how we are who we are, in a condition of
creaturely limits, dignifies us as human beings.

Even complaint is an expression out of dignity, reflecting a sense of self-worth. In Psalm 102, we hear complaint
that others fail to honor the psalmist's person and complaint of a pain that fractures not only physically and psychologically but also socially. "All day my enemies criticize
me. The ones who praised me curse against me," the
psalmist declares, showing a sense of self that incorporates a past when his reputation was good and people recognized him as a person of great worth. With the ravages
of pain and age, inseparable in this psalm, the psalmist has
lost his standing in the community. For this, the psalmist
blames God. "You have picked me up and tossed me
aside," an expression that underscores the elevation and

demotion that the psalmist has experienced within the community.

The psalmist's finitude and consequent imperfections and limitations predominate, in the first part of the psalm, as the source of great pain and grief. "Hurry, answer me," the psalmist cries, "for my days pass away like smoke." The undiscriminating transience created by fire provides apt similes for the psalmist's condition. He is wholly affected, from bones to heart/mind,[7] burned into a smoldering pile, withered like grass relentlessly stricken by the sun. The psalmist laments his failing condition and the pain and grief that accompany it. There is nothing romantic or lovely about this; it is anguished and heartbreaking. The psalmist's complaint is wholly human and reflects the most basic characteristic of what it means to be human.

That we are human as so noted, makes pain simply a part of what it means to be alive [. . .] and to die. "To be human, we must be finite in the whole of our existence."[8] Clearly these are not, as Sulmasy admits, pastoral conclusions that aim first to comfort and encourage; they are rather conclusions that reflect attempts to understand. What we do with them matters. Accepting one's creaturely, materialness does not mean that there is no place for protest against pain. Even in the context of the psalmist's recognition of the ongoing nature of humanity, that generations will succeed him, and that God goes on forever, the psalmist prays to live a full life — "do not bring me up with half my days." Being human, with its paradox of limitation and loft, of finitude and boundless dreams, lies at the foundation of Dylan Thomas' poetic counsel and appeal to his father, "Do not go gentle into that good night."

But the protest against death cannot be absolute. Death is not endlessly avoidable, nor always the enemy. There is a time, in the context of a finite life, to allow a space for death. Yet our culture is deeply committed to denying this, and we do so at great cost. Our commitment to keep people alive, no matter the conditions, their age, or even their wishes, is evident all around us. News reports are filled with information about how this or that illness can be averted or corrected by this or that medication, dietary change, or surgical procedure. I do not mean to suggest that efforts to ensure a full and healthy life are misplaced and that we should not employ the medical means available to us to enable such life. I mean simply to challenge the thinking that disallows any place for death, that demonstrates an inability to accept that our bodies are complex and wonderful organisms that simply cannot go on forever. Yet, "no one dies of old age, or so it would be legislated if actuaries ruled the world," Sherwin Nuland observes.[9] Although Nuland, a writer, surgeon, and professor of medicine at Yale University, notes, "I'm convinced that plenty of people do die of old age," a cause of death must be cited. "Everywhere in the world, it is illegal to die of old age."[10] Citing a cause is to identify the enemy. In such thinking, illness is an assault and death an enemy to be confronted and defeated.

Acknowledging and accepting what and who we are as human beings makes a place for pain, illness, and death. In the process, it changes the nature of questions of theodicy and may even render them moot. At the very least, it changes the tenor of the inquiry and disallows easy answers that depend finally on defining and defending ideas about what and who God is. We see such disruption of assumptions at the end of the biblical book of Job with its swift dismissal of particular answers and the introduction of a categorically different way of thinking. The narrator sets readers up at the beginning of the book to wonder about God's justification for Job's great suffering, and the poetic dialogues of Job and his friends that compose the majority of the text sustain the difficulty of these questions. When God finally speaks, readers expecting an answer are frustrated. Instead, God goes into great and magnificent detail about the makings and machinations of the world and its inhabitants; and Job's final words, in response to God, demonstrate a radically different way of thinking than what dominated in the preceding chapters. Job's final words do not reflect questions about whether or not Job deserved to suffer; instead, they have to do with who Job is. That the Hebrew of Job's speech is difficult to translate with a single sense and implication is telling. The most popular translation into English implies that Job regrets having said anything at all and resigns himself to being puny, ignorant, and insignificant, vis-à-vis a great (and bullying) God. However, the Hebrew also allows a translation flooded with a sense of satisfaction and comfort as Job finally comes to know what and who he is—a human being, paradoxically both little less than an angel and utterly dust. The voice of Psalm 102 similarly holds the particular value of an individual and his or her insignificance in the context of a wide world in productive tension to the end. Earnestly requesting that God not cut the psalmist's life too short, the psalmist also notes the incredible vastness of the earth and the heavens, the timeless nature of God, and the promise of future generations who will "abide" and "carry on."

Loosening Pain's Embrace

The sense of satisfaction and comfort that we may hear in Job's final words do not preclude the reality of his great suffering and the merit of his protest. In the book's epilogue, God commends Job, vindicating his questions, complaints, and challenges, while rebuking Job's friends who had tried to defend God against Job's accusations. The reality of Job's experience remains. The sense of satisfaction and comfort comes not because Job has forgotten or denied the experience of pain but through acknowledging and accepting exactly who he is, a human being imbued with freedom and an intrinsic dignity who is nevertheless finite in his creaturely materialness. Douglas Hoffman, whose research on the problems and possibilities of pain management has led to greater appreciation of the physiological effects of psychological processes, notes that to live an "authentic" life by acknowledging one's suffering as well as one's pleasures frequently undoes the pain that masks distress.[11]

The author of Psalm 102 cries bitterly out of the pain that he suffers and poignantly complains of wasting away in loneliness and distress. When the tone changes in the second part of the psalm, it is not because the psalmist's condition necessarily has improved. Rather, we find simply that the psalmist opens to the greater world and celebrates aspects of that world that underscore the paradoxes of human finitude and continuity, of pain and God's care for those suffering, of an imperfect world created by a perfect God. The psalmist loosens his embrace with pain and opens to appreciate other aspects of the reality of life. His perspective changes to acknowledge personal finitude in the context of the continuity of generations and the infinite nature of God. The psalmist's pain and earnest wish for his own full life are present in the second part of the psalm; but they do not override the sense that the world is populated by many others, now and in the future, who also are of concern to God. The psalmist notes that God listens to and helps those who suffer and that the community will continue in vitality and joy long after the psalmist is gone. The psalmist opens to others and loosens the grip on and of his own pain.

Stephen Levine writes of "softening around pain" in an effort to enable sufferers to relax. He has found that by accepting the condition of pain, people experience relief from it. He observes, "When pain arises in the body, it is very common to close around it. But our resistance and fear, our dread of the unpleasant, magnify pain. It is like closing your hand around a burning ember. The tighter you squeeze, the deeper you are seared."[12] Engaging mind and emotion as well as physiology, such softening results in a state of relaxation, which Levine reports eases pain for many people. Loosening their hold on pain loosens pain's hold on them. In Marni Jackson's pithy assessment, "Work against pain, and you lose. Work with pain, and the struggle lightens."[13] The psalmist's attention to others and the wider world in the second part of the psalm breathes more easily than his expressions of complaint in the first part. The strangling grasp of and with pain and the terror of his mortality give way to a widening embrace of all others and of the heavens and earth.

There is no reason to think that the psalmist's pain is gone in the second part of the psalm, but his attention is no longer focused on the anguish of his pain and anxiety of death. Instead, the psalmist has widened his attention to take in the whole world—from his community to the nations and "all the kings of the earth." The psalmist's scope includes generations to come, the diverse and distant nations, and the holiness and eternal nature of God. This great scope includes earth and heaven, the many and varied peoples that populate the world, and the sense of a God who is intimately associated with and different from the world. The psalmist takes special note of God's attention to those in pain and close to death. Loosening the tight embrace with pain, the psalmist looks to the whole world and meditates not only on how grand it is and that it will continue long after the psalmist is dead, but also that God goes on and in the going on continues to attend to those who suffer.

This attention to the world and its continuation reflects a loosening grip on the pain and a generous belief that God hears the cries of those in pain and helps them to experience their intrinsic liberty. The psalmist writes of a God worthy of praise because God hears the groans of the one who is bound, and "opens the ones dying."[14] Translations of this verse frequently emphasize an understanding of prisoners freed from a death-sentence, and the text indeed supports such a reading. However, the Hebrew also allows a more figurative interpretation in keeping with the psalms greater context, of an "opening to the pain" that brings relief/release. The process of opening about which Levine writes, and which weaves through his entire work, is a kind of acceptance of the condition of pain. People tell of feeling constricted and bound by their pain; when they begin to "soften" to it, to go into it and investigate, to be present to the pain in a way quite the opposite of distraction, Levine notes that it "[brings] a quietness to the mind" and enables them to go beyond the pain to inquire of the nature of their very selves.[15]

This self is not a closed, isolated, or radically independent entity, but is inextricably part of a much greater whole. In the process of softening to the pain, and opening up, Levine reports that sufferers tell of a new and welcome sense of space. "It is this willingness to play the edge of our pain that allows us a greater expansiveness, a deeper experience of who we really are. The resistance to pain obstructs the clear seeing of our true nature. Opening to our suffering we open to all."[16] The self-centered sentiments expressed at the beginning of the psalm give way to tell of others, of God, and of places and peoples near and far.

We see this transformation subtly in the conclusion of Earnest Gaines's novel, *A Lesson before Dying*, as a demonstration of one person's recovered humanity in the face of his death. A young, poor African American boy named Jefferson suffers the dehumanizing effects of racism. When Jefferson's godmother, Miss Emma, hears that he has been sentenced to death for a murder for which he may or may not have been responsible, she simply cannot accept the lawyer's dehumanizing dismissal of Jefferson as a "hog." The narrator, a schoolteacher named Grant, reluctantly agrees to his aunt's and Emma's request to make a man of Jefferson before Jefferson is killed. Although Jefferson's pain is not the pain of illness, his is a terminal condition. The turning-point in Jefferson's character seems to be his acceptance of responsibility for others, which demonstrates his full humanity. But that isn't all. At the urging of Grant, Jefferson keeps a journal before his execution, a journal that reveals new appreciation of a greater world and recognition of himself as a full human being:

> "day breakin sun comin up   the bird in the
> tre soun like a blu bird   sky blu blu mr
> wigin   good by mr wigin tell them im
> strong tell them im a man [. . .]." [17]

The new perspective that is gained by opening to the pain challenges impressions that one's pain and death distinguish oneself from others. The first part of the psalm, dominated by complaint, is also dominated by the psalmist's focus on himself. "I," "me," and/or "my" are present in every colon except one. The psalmist struggles for recognition of his personhood in the face of pain and death. To be human is to die, but the dying can be dehumanizing. Crying out of the failing of his body and the transience of his life, the psalmist finds that the most accurate descriptions of his condition come from the non-human world — "smoke," "a smoldering pile," "stricken grass," three kinds of birds, and drying vegetation. Appreciating the wider world and acknowledging that one is a part of it reshapes ideas of the self to allow that one's identity is wrapped up in a much greater whole. "We begin to stop thinking of these different qualities of mind as being 'I' and start to open to the space, the wholeness, within which the events are occurring: a nonjudging, exquisitely merciful space that we have access to in the heart, [. . .] the essence of mind itself [. . .] It is the root of that which we refer to when we say 'I am.'"[18]

However, even in the context of appreciating oneself as part of a greater whole, the reality of one's own pain and/or anxiety about one's own death remains. In the humorous words of "a Jewish Buddhist": If there is no self, then whose arthritis is this?[19] The psalmist continues throughout the psalm to express concern about the length of his particular life: "my days pass away like smoke," "my days are like a spreading shadow," and "My God, do not bring me up with only half my days." Even embedded in recognition of the greater world, of God's interest in the welfare of those who suffer, and of a people and God that will continue long after the psalmist has died, the psalmist still desires a full life, a longer life. The psalmist exclaims in the midst of eloquent appreciation of a wider world and generations that will succeed him, "[God] has broken my strength along the way; he has shortened my days." And in the face of God's eternal nature, "My God, do not bring me up with only half my days though your years are a generation of generations."

Statistics indicate that despite our wishes and efforts, most people experience great pain and indignity in the process of their dying. Loss of continence, the cruel tricks of dementia, the manner in which pain can warp a personality, are only a few of the ways that dying can compromise a person's sense of self. A "good death" has come to be associated with the maintenance of dignity. However, Nuland notes, "the belief in the probability of death with dignity is our, and society's, attempt to deal with the reality of what is all too frequently a series of destructive events that involve by their very nature the disintegration of the dying person's humanity. I have not often seen much dignity in the process by which we die."[20]

Similarly, Arthur Kleinman writes of an "embodied demoralization." "Technical rationality and technology of biomedicine" together with "the sentimentality and gratuitous optimism of Hollywood" deny the very real experience that some sufferers have of despair, great pain, and loss of dignity. An elderly woman with leukemia said to Kleinman, "Now its [sic] time to let me die on my terms [. . .] A psychiatrist told me I was depressed. Of course, I am. Isn't that what suffering is supposed to be? I want to bring it all to a close. Do I have to go with a smile on my face? That seems to me ridiculous, and insulting."[21]

Frequently the conditions of a person's dying are difficult and demeaning. The psalmist tells of great suffering in his dying and complains bitterly out of his anguish. In the process, he repeatedly notes the transient nature of his life. "My days are like a spreading shadow," the psalmist tells, "and I dry up like vegetation." Immediately following this expression of his end, the psalmist says, by way of contrast, "But you, God, dwell forever." This statement marks the turning-point of the psalmist's loosening embrace with pain as he opens to others and to the boundlessness of God. The author of Psalm 102 lives, in his attention to the greater world, with an eye toward his death. In doing so, the psalmist clings less tightly to his own pain and impending death; simultaneously, pain's grip on his suffering self loosens.

To Go Shining

Psalm 102 describes the indignity that can characterize a person's dying, and it models the frank acceptance of the limitations of an individual life in the context of a greater world. Psalm 102 does not conclude with fairy-tale resolution, but there is a sense of acceptance, of "bringing it all to a close" insofar as the psalmist removes himself from the final picture. The tone is not one of personal resignation or regret for what is not, but of an open-minded embrace of all that really is. Following an earnest request to be allowed to live his allotted lifetime, the psalmist looks to the earth and heavens in their dynamism and finitude, and wonders at the God whose "years will not be completed." The psalm ends with a statement that may be conjecture, wish, or optimism but is presented as a simple fact of the countless succession of new generations: "The children of your servants will abide, and their offspring will carry on before you." Finally, then, the psalmist notes continuity in the family of people.

The psalmist situates his dying in recognition of a greater world that goes on, in its impermanence and change, by the grace of God. Such recognition makes it possible to accept death as a "making room" for what continues, that it is necessary for some to die as others are born. This is not morbid or pessimistic but practical and realistic, and to the dying it may even be a comfort. According to Navajo legend, the purpose of death is to create space for the living: "If we all live and continue to increase as we have done in the past, the earth will be too small to hold us, and there will be no room for the corn-fields. It is better that each of us should live but a limited time on this earth, then leave and make room for the chil-dren."[22] The psalmist concentrates on all that is and all who are around him and without him, situating his indi-vidual self, which is in great pain and dying, in a greater whole that will continue after he is gone.

This perspective reflects a generosity and humbleness of heart that sees one's place as transitory. It is not belittling or dismissive of an individual's life, but honestly recog-nizes that no one person can be everything forever. In the words of humorist Garrison Keillor, "Nature doesn't care about your golden years; it's aiming for turnover."[23] Novelty enriches and energizes, and no matter how grand and large a life, there is a time for new life to take its place. Nuland notes that "there is a vanity in all of this [attempt-ing to prolong endlessly our lives], and it demeans us. [. . .] Far from being irreplaceable, we *should* be replaced."[24] This is not to reject attempts to provide cure and rehabili-tation; it is simply to advise exercising wisdom in making decisions so that a person's life not be prolonged for the sole reason of disallowing death. There is no perfect equa-tion for making appropriate decisions in such a context. However, we do well to keep in mind the danger of trying every possible means to keep ourselves or a loved one alive in cases in which "Persistence can only break the hearts of those we love and of ourselves as well, not to mention the purse of society that should be spent for the care of others who have not yet lived their allotted time."[25] The psalmist's attention turns from his own unique person to those who will succeed him—those who will survive him within the psalmist's community, populations across the world, and future generations. By opening up and "softening around" his pain and death, the psalmist looks out in love at place, people, and God.

In the face of our limits as human beings, limits that subject us to pain and finally death, the poet of Psalm 102 wonders at what is limitless. Marveling at the infinite nature of God, he reconciles what is particular and finite with what is without bounds. The psalmist brings the particularity of peoples, place, and even space, into the purview of a God deeply interested in the world and its inhabitants, telling that what goes on forever attends to what is bounded and constrained. The pain of the poor, those imprisoned, and the ones who are dying lies in the full and open gaze of the one who "established the surface of the earth, and made the heavens." The psalmist expresses awe at the mystery of a limitless God intimately involved in the limitations of the earth and those who live, suffer, delight, and die in it.

The psalmist's pain and the certainty of his death persist, suggested by the exclamation of "broken strength" and "shortened days." Yet they are embedded in wondered acknowledgement of the world and God's involvement in it. The psalmist recognizes that the world is much greater than his pain and wasting death. This recognition is accompanied by reassurance that an individual's pain is not thereby rendered unimportant or insignificant. On the contrary, it is the focus and priority of none other than the God of heaven and earth. But the psalmist reshapes ideas about his own impermanence to celebrate the succession of generations who abide in the care and keeping of God. In the process, the psalm witnesses to the love that God demonstrates by involvement in the world of impermanence, pain, and death despite being infinite and other. Love bridges the divide between what is finite and what is infinite, between what is limited and limitless, between people and God. "Only love has the infinite character that points beyond the finitude of the human condition."[26] Psalm 102 is a very human expression of what William May identifies in the biblical prophet Isaiah's unnamed "suffering servant." May writes that his suffering is "an attending to, a following, a tracking after the powerful will that creates, preserves, and upholds in love."[27]

The psalm moves from complaint to wonderment. In the process, readers witness dispassion for the one in pain/dying give way to a broad love expressed by that very person who is suffering. It is a love born of appreciation for and engagement in the context of his life—love of the psalmist for sacred place, his community, God, the wider world, and others imprisoned by pain. "The dignity that we seek in dying must be found in the dignity with which we have lived our lives.[. . .] The art of dying is the art of living. The honesty and grace of the years of life that are ending is the real measure of how we die."[28] The psalmist tenderly considers his community, treasuring the site that they associate with the presence, promise, and glory of God and marvels at the power and persistence of the Creator.

The psalmist's transformation in Psalm 102 is a kind of shining. From bitterness and grief at a body wasting away, long sleepless nights alone, and terrible contemplation of the brevity of his life, the psalmist turns to focus on the infinite nature of the world around him. This world that preceded his birth and will continue long after his death evokes in the psalm's second half reflective awe and praise for that which creates and sustains. Sometimes well-managed pain, without concern for addiction, in a chosen place surrounded by caring individuals, allows a dying person the possibility of such shining. This is how Marni Jackson describes her time caring for the dying "Carole."

"She seemed to have burned her way down through the usual resentments and fears to a light, titanium core of love."[29] Cicely Saunders developed the system of hospice care based on her medical training, listening to the wishes of those in great pain and dying, and compassionately considering the part that friends and family play in a person's final act. Kleinman writes of a 63-year-old college teacher dying from lung cancer who had hospice care before his death, care that allowed him to die as he wished. "Rather than having felt defeat, demoralization, or despair as the end approached; he felt remoralized. This sense of moral regeneration was so strong that in interviewing him just before he died, I, myself, caught it and felt uplifted by his spirit." Kleinman writes of "a sense of expansion, completion, even joyousness."[30]

The psalms do not definitively prescribe how people are to live or die but reflect how people have attempted not only to make sense of living and dying but also simply to express aspects of living and dying. Psalm 102 provides a window into an individual's life as he dies. In it, we see a person who has lived well and laments his degeneration. We hear a person who wonders in awe at the scope and diversity of the world, attention to those who suffer, and the continuity of human generations. "If this world is a place where we may learn of our involvement in immortal love, [. . .] such learning is only possible [. . .] because that love involves us so inescapably in the limits, sufferings, and sorrows of mortality."[31] The poet of Psalm 102 witnesses to a broad and embracing love, love of life and of the surrounding world, even, perhaps especially, in the condition of his death.

Conclusion

"We shall not cease from exploration
And the end of all our exploring
Will be to arrive where we started
And know the place for the first time." —*T. S. Eliot*

Although the presence and size of this book might suggest otherwise, I do not know much at all about pain. It is a huge problem, difficult to define, and hard to describe. Pain drives people to ask questions of meaning and their answers vary. I have sought, in the course of this book, to listen. In the process, I hope that readers have heard something new, something helpful in thinking about their own pain and/or the pain of others that may facilitate healing. Pain disintegrates a person, driving a wedge between a person's sense of body and self, and fracturing relationships, too; but it can also catalyze a process of integration whereby the whole of a person and his or her life comes together in an unprecedented manner. To date, there does not seem to be any one way to ensure the latter and minimize or obviate the former. They seem instead to be related, like the two sides of one coin, impossible to have one without the other. To *heal* is to make *whole*, and these words are etymologically related to the word *holy*.

217

Whatever one's faith tradition (or absence of it), the relationship of these words suggests that there is something sacred in the wholeness of a person, and that healing is the process of integrating experiences with characteristics (both external and internal), attitude, beliefs, and relationships into the warp and woof of a person's life.

There is no "life" except as it is lived, and the process of living is messy. Sometimes it is really hard. A person can be cured of pain; but for most people cure eludes, and pain's problems add up. To live through pain is to be fully alive as the unique person each of us is, even in the context of pain. It is to in-corpor-ate, into the multifaceted nature of our selves and the ways in which we are, the variety of experiences, good and bad, that we have and face. Living through pain involves recognizing that each of us is constantly changing, as are our circumstances, and embracing that dynamism is a part of what it means to be fully alive. Living through pain, then, involves recognizing the real conditions of one's life and self, and determining simply to be and do, in ever-changing circumstances, as fully as possible.

Such recognition does not mean that a person assume the silent suffering of a righteous martyr. On the contrary, such recognition often leads to gut-wrenching cries of heartfelt complaint. The psalmists dignify the place of complaint and strident cry out of conditions that seem unbearable. They do not model super-human endurance and cheer in terrific suffering. Neither do they tell how a person can be healed through complaint, or through silent suffering, for that matter. However, they do give voice to conditions that may seem inexpressibly terrible, and they articulate the kinds of theologically challenging questions that a suffering person may hesitate to ask out loud. Furthermore, they tell how influential the relationship of others to the person in pain can be, both in terms of how others' behavior affects for good and ill the pain of the sufferer, as well as the sufferer's subjectivity vis-à-vis others. Finally, each psalm also supposes the intrinsic value of the person in pain, justified in telling his or her experience no matter how fraught with questions, problematic implications, and despair. The sufferer warrants attention and claims a hearing, these psalms suggest. Sometimes the telling itself facilitates healing.

Pain is baffling and frequently frustrating. Different for each person and varying within each case, no single treatment can be applied with consistent success. In this book, I have come no closer to defining or describing pain than I considered at the beginning; neither have I discovered and revealed a "magic bullet" to kill pain. Although the starting point for my inquiry was physical pain, pain is a whole person event. Therefore, talking about chronic physical pain inevitably leads to its emotional, psychological, spiritual, and social effects. Appreciating this further complicates our understanding of pain as we find that social rejection, financial insecurity, professional failure, and fractured relationships are themselves painful and frequently inseparable from persistent headache or backache. Our meditation on problems with pain, the meanings that people seek and make of their pain, and the manner in which psalmists express aspects of pain, reflect that pain is a part of every person's life experience in some time, form, or fashion. The challenge then becomes how to deal with it, to acknowledge the reality of the experience, and in-corpor-ate it into one's life with healing.

There is no single way to do this; yet the *process* is its own success as much as or more than any conclusion or final result. The psalms that we considered here do not demonstrate a linear process, repeated and reinforced by each psalm. Instead, they witness to different aspects of the experience and to the challenges, frustrations, surprises, and glimpses of relief that accompany the journey through pain. Together, they tell a variety of responses to and interpretations of the experience of pain. I arranged our reading of them not to impose a definite succession of stages, but to invite readers to consider some aspects of a process of living through pain. Much of what we read is simply speaking out of pain, telling the terror, disappointments, and worries that the psalmists confront. Along the way, questions such as why the pain, and why me? emerge in a variety of ways; and the psalmists deal with the implications of their pain for relationships—with God, with other people, and in the context of a wider world.

These questions and the manner in which pain affects relationships (and vice versa) are timeless. That is, no matter a person's time or place, to ask such questions when faced with intractable pain is simply human. Appreciating that pain drives people to ask for meaning, we considered in chapter 2 and again in some of the psalms the ways in which people seek to make sense of their pain. Answers to the why questions vary, but all represent efforts to incorporate the pain into a person's life. That is, they all are a product of the search for wholeness. Observing the movement of ideas and the dynamic of experience in the psalms, we are reminded that answers to the why questions need not be static; and sometimes, the question of meaning itself becomes moot. For example, we observed development from an idea of pain as punishment to the sense that any person can nevertheless cry out of such pain for relief [. . .] even cry to the very God who that person thinks is punishing him or her. The movement itself suggests that the sufferer, whatever may be his or her crime, can nevertheless seek to be relieved of pain and hope for comfort and compassion from those around him or her. In keeping with this observation, it is notable that God never makes such declarations in these psalms. Instead, while the psalmists wrestle with ideas of pain as God's punishment, they nevertheless also presume that their God is a God of help and healing, especially concerned with those who are in pain. It is likewise notable that although some of the psalmists suggest that they may have committed a crime deserving of punishment, which they may think their pain represents, such judgment of another's pain is never portrayed as appropriate. On the contrary, we discover that many psalmists identify egregious wrongdoing precisely in such judgment of pain by other people. The psalms instead suggest that the role of others vis-à-vis the person in pain should be one of listening, comforting, and seeking healing for the sufferer.

Healing is impossible without full recognition of the very real circumstances of that particular moment. In other words, to put it negatively, healing is impossible if one or another facet of one's experience and/or self is consistently denied. In the case of chronic pain, healing requires recognizing that pain has taken up residence. Consequently, it also requires recognizing how the pain is affecting one's life; and such acknowledgment allows that pain can change. Psalm 69 begins with a poignant cry acknowledging pain's presence and effect. The psalmist finds that attempts to stave off terrific trouble are futile, and she cries out that she is overwhelmed. "The waters have come in to my very self." There is no denying the pain. Her language is lament, complaint to God of the unfairness of it all, of a self come undone, of rejection, and being the subject of malicious gossip by others.

We observed in reading Psalm 69 a process of interpretation whereby earlier conclusions are challenged and either complicated or replaced. The psalmist's prayer is for attention and help, for rescue from the metaphorical waves of destructive pain that threaten to drown the psalmist. Matters of innocence and guilt are secondary to the psalmist's distress, yet the rumors, scorn, and even attack of others based on presumptions about the psalmist's guilt compound her pain. The psalmist describes such behavior by others as an affront not only to her but also to God. Instead of suffering on account of wrong-doing, the psalmist tells of suffering on account of God and expresses concern that others like her might likewise suffer.

Psalm 69 undercuts easy answers to the problem of pain, demonstrating instead a process of interpretation and finally confidence that even in the face of intractable pain, the sufferer is not alone and ignored but recognized and valued as a whole person, even with the pain. The matter of meaning, of determining reasons for the psalmist's pain, is a dominant theme and concludes with concern for others who suffer similarly. The psalmist's pain finally assumes meaning in being for others. The psalmist does not declare that her pain has been cured, but her exclamation that goodness infuses even the waters that had earlier proved an apt metaphor for distress demonstrates the integration of her experiences and how questions about reason and purpose are recast in confidence and hope.

The matter of pain as deserved punishment, undercut within Psalm 69 and reversed by its author to condemn the condemnation by others, is a dominant theme also in Psalm 38. By contrast with Psalm 69, the author of Psalm 38 identifies in his pain a punishment for wrong action. Instead, however, of simply complaining that he is miserable, the psalmist goes into notable detail about the kind and extent of his pain and expresses confidence that God is aware of it all. In such a context, the psalmist subtly does something remarkable: without denying his wrong-doing, he nevertheless expresses confidence in God's attention and assumes that God will help him. In other words, the psalmist does not accept his great pain as a burden to be born on account of earlier wrongdoing, but cries out for relief. Furthermore, the psalmist complains of people who ostracize him and seek to hurt him even more, identifying them as contributing to his pain. Despite earlier wrongdoing, the psalmist seeks to do good and complains that he is repaid with hatred and enmity. The psalmist's last words are a cry that God be near and help — a remarkable conclusion for this psalm that began with such clear association of pain with punishment.

Psalm 38 invites readers to move with the psalmist through a process that begins by interpreting pain as punishment for wrongdoing, then noting the destructive nature of pain, and finally declaring justification for seeking relief. Psalm 38 also invites readers to see with the psalmist how the behavior of others can inappropriately exacerbate the pain, suggesting that whatever an individual's interpretation of his or her pain, it is wrong for others to make such judgments and consequently to ignore and/or disparage the person in pain. In this psalm, we observe that whatever the reason for pain, pain's destructive nature is itself evil, accomplishing nothing beneficial. Consequently, the psalmist suggests that even in the face of a punishing pain, God is interested in its relief.

Sometimes the extent and duration of pain is so great that a person despairs of having any relief. No one can help; the sufferer is alone with pain and worn out from the struggle. In such a condition, a person of faith naturally questions God's interest, even presence at all. These are the conditions we hear in the voice of Psalm 88. In considering this most dark of the psalms, we observed that the psalmist's attitude is not transformed and expressed in relief or hope. Instead, the psalm actually ends with darkness. Psalm 88 is discomforting in its unabashed complaint of a condition out of which the psalmist sees no resolution, no chance of healing. It is the voice of one who feels on the cusp of death and yet for whom death does not come. This is not the psalm of one who believes, "God would not give me more than I can handle." This is the psalm of one who cries, "I can no more." The psalm is saturated with dark despair. Even human relationships, friends and family, do no good; and God seems utterly disinterested. Attention on God is sustained throughout and it resonates with the tone of one deeply betrayed.

That such a psalm is included in biblical texts may seem scandalous. Its presence, however, gives voice to what many people find to be the very real circumstances of their pain, undercutting a too easy theology and validating the hard questions that come with great suffering. The psalm does not resolve with expressions of thanksgiving or hope. It ends with *darkness*. Yet this final word, we observed, may paradoxically hint of light. That is, the condition of descending and inhabiting these darkest of depths may allow a radically new experience of life. The mystics propose that in this condition of losing everything, including a sense of direction or even hope, God's supportive presence is closest; the darkness is simply the blinding light of God. Whatever the case, Psalm 88 ends with darkness.

Psalm 22 begins with dark despair, including a sense of abandonment by God such as Psalm 88 described. However, within Psalm 22, we witness movement from such a condition, through trials and tribulations, to awe and thanksgiving. In reading it, we compared the progress of the psalmist to that of Joseph Campbell's archetypal "hero's journey." The psalmist is forced to make his way, shorn of every support, through territory populated by threatening beasts and terrifying circumstances. Suffering within and without, the psalmist feels less than human. Yet he is human, and this makes his journey especially powerful both for the community to which he returns, changed, and for readers of the psalm. The psalmist returns to his community with new insights to share and a message of courage and hope that is powerful precisely because of his humanity and what he has endured. The psalmist does not tell of being cured from his pain; but readers witness his healing. The sufferer integrates his experience of pain into the whole of his life. Rejoining his community is a crucial part of this integration, as is his willingness to declare that help is present in all places. The psalmist's concluding message is partly communicated simply by his stance within the human community. Furthermore, his declaration of God's attention to those in pain and of God's universality effectively tells the unity of all people. The psalmist integrates his experience of great pain and suffering into who he is and how he is, in order to bring a message of unity and hope back to others.

While the author of Psalm 22 integrates his experience of pain to tell of help and hope, the poet of Psalm 6 integrates her experience of pain to reject whatever prevents growth and development. After terrors and great suffering, the voice of Psalm 22 delivers an inclusive and welcome message to others. The author of Psalm 6 also suffers a compromising pain that disintegrates her; but in contrast to Psalm 22, when she speaks it is to *speak out against* prohibitive and destructive forces. In considering Psalm 6, we noted how the speaker begins with complaint of a pain that may or may not be justified as punishment.

The psalmist goes on simply to tell how destructive the pain is and consequently how justified the psalmist is in asking for relief. Exhausted and unrelieved, the psalmist weeps. The experience of such disintegrating pain is an experience of great loss, and the psalmist responds with grief. We observed, however, that after mourning, the psalmist turns with renewed energy and power against whomever or whatever causes her trouble and holds her back. The psalm ends with confidence that the psalmist will be vindicated, and whatever or whoever contributed to her suffering will be rebuffed and shamed.

The last of the psalms that we read in detail concerns death. In Psalm 102, we listened to the voice of one whose days are passing quickly away in a condition of frailty and loneliness. The psalmist complains that he is withering away, without either appetite or sleep. Those who once looked up to him now criticize him; even God, who once elevated the psalmist, now disregards him. The psalmist's pain is inseparable from deep sorrow at the transience of his life, until his perspective alters; then he wonders at the comparable infinity of God. Turning to contemplate his community and the wide world, the psalmist's tone changes from the complaint and sorrow of his pain and impending death, to awe and appreciation of God's unending nature and the continuity of generations. The psalmist notes that people suffering as he does are not without attention, and God "opens" those bound in the grip of pain and death. Although he does not cease wanting a full and long life, the psalmist's concern becomes instead appreciation of the earth and heavens, that they go on as does God whose "years will not be completed" and as does a community whose children "will abide, and their offspring carry on before you."

God never speaks in these psalms. Maybe God is as dumbfounded by the problem of pain as we are. Maybe God's silence represents the powerful expression of attentive listening. Some psalms tell as much; but some psalmists complain that God's *in*attention actually is the most painful thing about their condition. Explaining why represents a weak argument from silence. Without God's speech to confirm or deny the psalmist's complaints, worries, judgments, and hope, we are left with pain as a human issue. This goes both ways. That is, it has implications both for how others treat a person in pain and for how the person in pain acts in relation to the community.

Concerning the former, most of the psalms that we considered complain about the manner in which others' words and actions contributed to their pain. In reading Psalm 69, we observed that even though the psalmist does not claim to be innocent in all ways, she does claim to be innocent of the charges that others bring against her on account of her pain. Others had concluded that her pain was simply punishment for some wrongdoing and proceeded to treat her accordingly, with scorn and contempt. The psalmist's vitriolic response suggests that such treatment by others of the person in pain itself warrants punishment. That is, not only is such reactive judgment inappropriate, but also is itself a crime. Even in the case of pain that the psalmist considers to be deserved (as in the case of Psalm 38), the psalmist tells that the appropriate response of others should be to be near, to listen, to support, and to encourage. In telling this, the psalmist underscores her conclusion that the pain she suffers is finally simply destructive, justifying her prayer for company and help.

The psalmists also give to others, not in spite of their pain, but out of the context of their pain. Within these psalms we read of concern for others who are similar to the suffering psalmist and so vulnerable to the same pain (e.g. Psalm 69), of valuable lessons learned and testimony shared about goodness inherent in the world (e.g. Psalm 22), and of a person's intrinsic value, worthy of attention, and not compromised by pain (e.g. Psalm 102). The psalms themselves are contributions of persons in pain to others. They are the public words of pained persons, delivered with sometimes disturbing candor, poignantly demonstrating efforts to integrate the experience of terrific and intractable pain into the whole of a person's life.

Despite pain's particularity, and despite the singular nature of each of the biblical psalms, commonalities among the psalms exist, and these commonalities are revealing about the experience of pain. Each psalm speaks of a condition of systemic pain. The psalmist tells of suffering that is physical, but that also includes psychological and emotional distress, and has spiritual implications as well as a profound social dimension. In other words, every psalm tells of pain as a whole person problem. Every psalm also tells of the condition as a changing one. In no case is the experience static. Neither do we read a final conclusion or answer for the psalmist's pain. Instead, the psalmists move through their pain. The experience itself and its management is a dynamic process, as portrayed in these texts. However, within each psalm, and taken together, there is a sense that this process is not linear and predictable; rather, it meanders and branches off in directions different for each person. I have chosen psalms that represent various aspects of the experience of pain, and I have organized our discussion of them to demonstrate this non-linear, sometimes messy process of acknowledging and seeking to manage pain. In the process of this book, then, I hope to facilitate the search to incorporate the experience of pain into the whole of a person's life, allowing personal expression and development in keeping with the integrity of an individual connected to family, friends, and the greater community.

The psalmists do not assume that their faith will spare them pain; rather, out of their faith, they tell an ongoing process of integrating oneself and one's pain into a life fully lived. In many cases, the psalmists express a sense of hope and relief but say nothing of cure. Although several tell of God's attention and concern for the person suffering, they do not presume that God will take away the pain. Neither, however, do the psalmists suffer in silence; on the contrary, these psalms are themselves the speech of persons in pain who want relief. They consider that relief, however, in terms of presence and attention (God's and others') and suggest that also in the telling itself there is relief.

This book concerns pain, not simply as an object of intellectual scrutiny, but as a visceral experience that is at once both difficult to tell and demands a hearing. The ancient, biblical collection of psalms includes the voices of people speaking out of this experience in a variety of ways. Asking about pain and listening to the candid manner in which these ancient poets tell their stories gives us occasion to reflect on our own experiences of pain. It enriches our vocabulary and grammar for the expression and management of pain in an effort to *live through* pain, not simply to endure it or even to live in spite of it, but to live as a whole person even in the midst of pain.

By wrapping the pain into one's whole life, the pain itself is transformed. Meditating on such a possibility, Rachel Naomi Remen tells the process that yields an oyster's pearl. Although its shell protects an oyster's soft and tender body, its life requires that the oyster make itself vulnerable to injury and pain. It must open its shell to breathe, so sometimes a grain of sand gets inside. "Such grains of sand cause pain," Remen observes, "but an oyster does not alter its soft nature because of this [. . .] But it does respond. Slowly and patiently, the oyster wraps the grain of sand in thin translucent layers until, over time, it has created something of great value in the place where it was most vulnerable to pain."[1] We cannot live fully without risking the pain of injury and loss. Our challenge, then, is tenderly and patiently to wrap the pain into a life made richer and more beautiful not for the pain itself but for the process of our response to it.

Psalms Translations

Psalm 6

v.1 For the leader, on stringed instruments, according to the Eighth. A psalm of David:

YHWH, do not discipline me in your wrath,
    do not chasten me in your rage.

v.2 Be gracious to me, YHWH, for I am feeble.
    Heal me, YHWH, for my bones are shaking.

v.3 My whole self is terribly shaken,
    and you, YHWH—how long?

v.4 Return, YHWH, draw out my life
    deliver me on account of your kindness

v.5 For there is no remembrance of you in death,
    in Sheol, who gives thanks to you?

v.6 I am weary with my moaning,
    every night I soak my sleeping place with tears
    and dissolve my sick-bed.

v.7 My eye darkens from vexation,
    worn out by all those who hold me back.

v.8 Turn away from me all you troublemakers,
    for YHWH hears the sound of my crying

v.9 YHWH hears my supplication,
    YHWH accepts my prayer.

v.10 My enemies will be ashamed and shake greatly with terror,
    they will turn back, in a moment, they will be ashamed.

Psalm 22

> *v. 1 To the choirmaster, according to "the doe of the dawn."*
> *A psalm of David:*

My God, my God, why have you abandoned me?
  Far from my salvation, the sounds of my groaning.
v.2 My God, I call out by day, but you do not answer
  And at night, but I have no rest.
v.3 Yet you are holy, dwelling on the praises of Israel.
v.4 In you our ancestors trusted,
  They trusted and you rescued them.
v.5 To you they cried out and were delivered.
  In you they trusted and were not embarrassed.
v.6 But I am a worm and not a man,
  A joke of a human being and disdain of a people.
v.7 All who see me make fun of me.
  They gape and shake their heads.
v.8 "Go to YHWH. He will rescue him
  He will deliver him because he delights in him."
v.9 Indeed you drew me out from the belly,
  made me secure on my mother's breasts
v.10 On you I was cast from the womb.
  From my mother's belly, you have been my God.
v.11 Do not be distant from me
  for trouble is near and there is no help.
v.12 Many bulls encircle me,
  mighty ones from Bashan surround me.
v.13 They open their mouths against me,
  a preying, snarling lion.
v.14 I am poured out like water, all my bones are disjointed,
  my heart is like wax, melting in my guts.
v.15 My strength is dried up like a potsherd,
  and my tongue sticks in my jaws.
  You assigned me to the dust of death.
v.16 Dogs surround me, a wicked pack.
  Like a lion they circumscribe my hands and feet.
v.17 I count all my bones.
  They, they watch and stare at me.

v.18 They divide my garments among them
    And over my clothes they cast lots.

v.19 But you, YHWH, do not be far off,
    my aid, hurry to my help.

v.20 Deliver my self away from the sword
    from the power of the dog, just me.

v.21 Save me from the lion's mouth.
    From the horns of the wild ox, answer me.

v.22 I will recount your name to my brothers,
    in the midst of the assembly I will praise you.

v.23 You who fear/respect YHWH, praise him.
    All of Jacob's descendants, honor him.
    Stand in awe of him, all Israel's descendants.

v.24 For God did not disdain or abhor the affliction of the
        afflicted
    nor did God hide God's face from him,
    and when he cried out to God, he heard.

v.25 On account of you is my praise in the great
        congregation,
    I will make good my vows before those who fear him.

v.26 The afflicted shall eat and be satisfied,
    those who seek YHWH shall praise him.
    May your heart live forever!

v.27 All the ends of the earth shall remember and return to
        YHWH,
    all the families of the nations shall bow down before
        you.

v.28 For the kingship is YHWH's,
    and he reigns over nations.

v.29 All the fat of the earth shall eat and bow down,
    all those who go down to the dust shall kneel before
        him,
    and whose spirit is not vibrant.

v.30 Offspring shall serve him,
    future generations will hear of the Lord.

v.31 They will go in and relate his righteousness,
    to a people (un)born, what he has done.

Psalm 38

v. 1 A psalm of David, to remind:
YHWH, do not rebuke me in your wrath
    nor chasten me in your rage.
v.2 For your arrows have sunk into me,
    and your hand has descended on me.
v.3 There is no soundness in my flesh because of your
        indignation,
    there is no wholeness/shalom in my bones because of
      my sin.
v.4 For my wrongdoings have gone over my head,
    like a weighty burden, too weighty for me.
v.5 My wounds stink and rot because of my foolishness.
v.6 I am exceedingly twisted and bent.
    All day long I walk around gloomy.
v.7 For my loins are full of burning,
    and there is no soundness in my flesh.
v.8 I am exceedingly numbed and crushed,
    I howl from the groaning of my heart.
v.9 O Lord, all my longing is before you,
    and my sighing is not hidden from you.
v. 10 My mind reels, my strength fails me,
    and the light of my eyes, even they—there is nothing
    with me.
v.11 My lovers and friends stand aloof from my injury,
    those closest to me stand far away.
v.12 Those who seek my life strike out,
    those who want to hurt me speak malice,
    they ponder treachery all the time.
v.13 But I am like the deaf, I do not hear;
    and like the dumb, I don't open my mouth.
v.14 I am like a man who does not hear,
    and there is no retort in his mouth.
v.15 But for you, YHWH, I wait;
    you, you will answer, my Lord, my God
v.16 When I say, "lest they laugh at me,
    or when my foot slips, gloat over me."

v.17 For I am ready to stumble,
    my pain is continually before me.
v.18 I confess my iniquity,
    I am sorry about my sin.
v.19 And my mortal enemies are vast,
    many are those who wrongly hate me.
v.20 Those who repay evil for good
    harass me on account of my pursuing good.
v.21 Do not leave me, YHWH my God,
    Do not be far from me.
v.22 Hurry to my aid, my Lord, my salvation.

Psalm 69

v.1   To the leader, according to the Lilies, of David:
Save me, O God,
    for the waters have come in to my very self.
v.2 I have sunk in the mire of the deeps,
    and there is no place to stand;
  I have come in to the depths of the water,
    and rushing streams dashed over me.
v.3 I am exhausted from calling out,
    my throat is parched.
   My eyes are done,
    waiting for my God.
v.4 Many more than the hairs on my head are those who
        hate me for no reason.
    Vast are those who would annihilate me, my deceitful
        enemies.
    Should I give back what I have not robbed?
v.5 O God, you know my folly,
    and my wrongdoing is not concealed from you.
v.6 Do not let those who hope in you be shamed
        of/on account of me
    O Lord, YHWH of hosts
  Do not let those who seek you be humiliated because of
        me,
    O God of Israel.

v.7 Because on account of you I have put up with scorn.
     Insult covers my face.

v.8 I have become estranged from my brothers,
     alienated from my mother's children.

v.9 Because passion for your house consumed me,
     The scorn of those who scorned you fell on me.

v.10 I wept with the fasting of my soul,
     and I was scorned for it.

v.11 I made sackcloth my clothing,
     and I became an allegory for them.

v.12 Those who sit in the gate opine about me,
     and drunkards make up ditties about me.

v.13 But I, my prayer is for you, O YHWH.
     At the right time, in your abundant kindness,
     answer me with the surety of your salvation.

v.14 Rescue me from the mud and do not let me sink.
     Let me be rescued from those who hate me.
     and from the depths of the waters.

v.15 Do not let the rushing streams of water dash over me,
     and do not let the deeps swallow me up,
     nor the Pit close its mouth on me.

v.16 Answer me, YHWH, for your kindness is good,
     according to your abundant compassion, turn to me.

v.17 Do not hide your face from your servant,
     for I am in distress.
     Hurry, answer me.

v.18 Come close to my self, rescue it.
     On account of my enemies, ransom me.

v.19 You know my scorn, my shame, and my ignominy,
     All my foes are before you.

v.20 Scorn has broken my heart, I am sick.
     I waited for pity but there wasn't any,
     for comforters, but found none.

v.21 They gave for my food/hunger bitter poison/gall,
     and for my thirst vinegar to drink.

v.22 Let their table be a snare for them,
     a lure for their allies.

v.23 Make their eyes too dim to see,
     and their loins continually tremble.
v.24 Pour out your indignation on them,
     and your burning anger overtake them.
v.25 May their encampment be desolate,
     let no one live in their tents.
v.26 Because you, whomever you have struck, they pursue,
     and the pain of your stabbings they recount.
v.27 Add guilt to their guilt,
     and do not let them into your righteousness.
v.28 Let them be wiped out from the book of the living,
     do not let them be written with the righteous ones.
v.29 But I am afflicted and in pain.
     Your salvation, O God, sets me up high.
v.30 I will praise the name of God with song,
     I will magnify him with thanksgiving.
v.31 It is better to YHWH than an ox or a bull with horn
     and hooves.
v.32 The afflicted will see, they will rejoice.
     Those who seek God, let your hearts live.
v.33 For YHWH listens to the needy,
     and he does not despise (his) prisoners.
v.34 The heavens and the earth will praise him,
     the seas and all that moves about in them.
v.35 For God will save Zion and (re)build the cities of
     Judah,
     and they will return there and inherit it.
v.36 The children of his servants will possess it,
     and those who love his name will dwell in it.

Psalm 88

v.1 A psalm, a Korahthite melody for the leader on mahalath lean-noth. A maskil of Heman the Ezrahite.
YHWH, God of my salvation,
     I cry out by day, by night in your presence.
v.2 Let my prayer come in before you,
     incline your ear to my ringing cry.

v.3 My self is full of troubles,
    my life is on the brink of the land of the dead.
v.4 I am considered with those going down to the Pit,
    I am like a strongman for whom there is no help.
v.5 With the dead, released; like the slain grave-dwellers
    whom you no longer remember, cut off from your
        hand.
v.6 You put me in the bottom of the Pit,
    in dark places, in the deeps.
v.7 Your rage lies heavy on me,
    you overwhelm me with all your breakers.

Selah

v.8 You distanced those known to me,
    You set me up as an abomination to them,
    Spent. And I do not go out.
v.9 My eye tires from my affliction,
    I called out to you, YHWH, every day, I spread out my
        hands.
v.10 Do you work wonders for the dead?
    Or the ghosts rise up to thank you?

Selah

v.11 Is your kindness recounted in the grave?
    Your loyalty in the place of ruin?
v.12 Is your wonder known in the darkness?
    Or your righteousness in the land of oblivion?
v.13 But I, I cry for help to you, O YHWH,
    In the morning my prayer greets you.
v.14 Why, YHWH, do you spurn my self,
    do you hide your face from me?
v.15 I have been afflicted and close to death from my youth.
    I endure your terrors. I despair.
v.16 Your wrath has swept over me,
    your alarms destroy me.
v.17 They surround me like water every day
    they close in over me.
v.18 You distanced lover and friend from me,
    The ones known to me, —darkness.

Psalm 102

v.1 A prayer of someone afflicted when he is feeble and he pours out his complaint before YHWH.

O YHWH, hear my prayer
> and let my cry for help come in to you.

v.2 Do not hide your face from me on the day of my
> distress,
>> incline your ear to me on the day when I call out.
>> Hurry, answer me.

v.3 For my days pass away like smoke,
> and my bones burn like a smoldering pile.

v.4 My heart withers like stricken grass
> because I forget to eat my food.

v.5 With the sound of my moaning,
> and my bones clinging to my flesh,

v.6 I resemble a Kaath-bird of the wilderness.
> I am like an owl of the ruins.

v.7 I lie awake
> and am like a lone bird on a roof.

v.8 All day my enemies criticize me.
> The ones who praised me curse against me

v.9 For I eat ashes like bread
> and into my drink I stir my tears,

v.10 Because of your indignation and wrath.
> For you have picked me up and tossed me aside.

v.11 My days are like a spreading shadow,
> and I dry up like vegetation.

v.12 But you YHWH dwell forever,
> and your memorial from generation to generation.

v.13 You will rise up and have compassion on Zion,
> for it is time to show favor to her,
> the appointed time has come.

v.14 For your servants are pleased with her stones,
> and favor her dust.

v.15 The nations will fear the name of YHWH,
> and all the kings of the earth, your glory.

v.16 For YHWH built Zion,
> he appeared in his glory.

v.17 He turned to the prayer of the destitute,
   he did not despise their prayer.

v.18 This was written for the next generation,
   And a people to be created will praise Yah

v.19 (For YHWH overlooked his holy place,
   from heaven to earth he looked.

v.20 To hear the prisoner's groan,
   to open the ones dying.)

v.21 To recount in Zion the name of YHWH,
   and his praise-psalm in Jerusalem,

v.22 When the peoples are gathered together
   and kingdoms to worship YHWH.

v.23 He has broken my strength along the way,
   he has shortened my days.

v.24 "My God," I say, "do not bring me up with only half
     my days
   though your years are a generation of generations.

v.25 You established the surface of the earth,
   and your hands made the heavens.

v.26 They perish, but you remain forever.
   All of them will wear out like a garment.
   You change them like clothes and they change.

v.27 But you are he,
   and your years will not be completed.

v.28 The children of your servants will abide,
   and their offspring will carry on before you."

Notes

✎

Notes to Introduction

1. The actual duration of suffering is less helpful in defining pain as "chronic" (versus "acute") than the simple sense of pain that defies relief. Acute pain, such as one might experience with a definable injury that progresses immediately toward healing, may also affect a person completely; but it does so less consistently and profoundly than chronic pain.

2. In this way pain is like porn. Readers may remember the words of Justice Potter Stewart in the case of Jacobellis versus Ohio concerning the definition of "hard-core pornography." He famously noted, "I shall not today attempt further to define the kinds of material I understand to be embraced within that shorthand description; and perhaps I could never succeed in intelligibly doing so. *But I know it when I see it,* and the motion picture involved in this case is not that." (378 U.S. 184 [1964], italics mine).

3. The *psalms* are individual poetic units/songs within the collection titled *Psalms*; *psalmist* is a term denoting the author(s) of a psalm.

4. Harold S. Kushner's slim volume, *When Bad Things Happen to Good People* (New York: Schocken Books, 1981; repr. New York: Avon Books, 1983) wrestles well with these same issues in a manner very much in keeping with the psalms. Page references are to the 1983 edition.

5. David Morris composed a book-length study showing how our cultural milieu informs our experience of pain in *The Culture of Pain* (Berkeley: University of California Press, 1993).

241

6. Rachel Naomi Remen makes such an observation after hearing a Native American, Episcopal bishop explain a Navaho Christology: "This man Jesus, He is good medicine." (*My Grandfather's Blessings: Stories of Strength, Refuge, and Belonging* [New York: Riverhead Books, 2000], 100). Remen is a clinical professor of family and community medicine at the University of California in San Francisco. She cofounded and directs the Commonweal Cancer Help Program in Bolinas, California.

7. Rachel Naomi Remen's books cite numerous real cases of such conditions. Furthermore, she notes that some very sick and pained patients report discovering a feeling of healthiness that they never had before the onset of injury or illness and before engaging the process of coming to terms with their whole selves in present conditions. See especially *Kitchen Table Wisdom: Stories that Heal* (New York: Riverhead Books, 1996), and *My Grandfather's Blessings.*

Notes to Chapter 1

1. I borrow David B. Morris's terminology to describe that at the foundation of the problem of defining pain is a contemporary understanding of the self as divisible into physical and mental. See Morris, *Culture of Pain.*

2. "Former HHS Secretary Sullivan, Former Surgeon General Satcher Announce Educational Tool to Fight 'Epidemic' of Untreated Pain," *US Newswire* via COMTEX (September 8, 2003).

3. Walter F. Stewart, Judith A. Ricci, Elsbeth Chee, David Morganstein, and Richard Lipton, "Lost Productive Time and Cost Due to Common Pain Conditions in the US Workforce," *JAMA* 290 (2003): 2443–2454.

4. Stewart, et al., "Lost Productive Time," 2443.

5. Maryann S. Bates, *Biocultural Dimensions of Chronic Pain: Implications for Treatment of Multi-ethnic Populations*, SUNY Series in Medical Anthropology (Albany: State University of New York Press, 1996), xv.

6. Dennis C. Turk, "Assess the Person, Not Just the Pain," n.p. *Pain: Clinical Updates 1* (September 1993). http://www.iasp-pain.org/PCU93c.html (accessed July 19, 2003). Dr. Turk of the Pain Evaluation and Treatment Institute at the University of Pittsburgh School of Medicine is one of the leading researchers of pain and its management, collaborating with Ronald Melzack (one of the first to address pain as a legitimate medical problem of its own) in the *Handbook of Pain Assessment* (New York: Guilford

Press, 1992), an oft-cited tool in medical and related research on pain.

7. Personal conversation, August 2004. Dr. Cifu is the chair of the Department of Physical Medicine and Rehabilitation at Virginia Commonwealth University, a *US News and World Report* Top 20 Rehabilitation program.

8. R. L. Robinson, et al., "Economic Cost and Epidemiological Characteristics of Patients with Fibromyalgia Claims," *Journal of Rheumatology* 30 (2003): 1318–1325.

9. Steven F. Brena, *Chronic Pain: America's Hidden Epidemic* (New York: Atheneum/SMI, 1978).

10. Kathryn Weiner, "Pain is an Epidemic" (AAPM Special Message), 2002.

11. The results of the survey are available at http://www.chiro.org/LINKS/FULL/1999_National_Pain_Survey.html (accessed May 12, 2003).

12. Robert Dallek, "The Medical Ordeals of JFK," *Atlantic Monthly* 290 (December 2002): 49–52, 54f.

13. Ronald Melzack and Patrick D. Wall, *The Challenge of Pain* (New York: Penguin, 1982), 267. This book was first published as *The Puzzle of Pain* in 1973.

14. Individual physicians, multidisciplinary pain clinics, and a variety of groups defined by addressing the problem of pain provide good sources of information about medical treatment options. Among many sources of information and commentary on issues of access to pain treatment is an excellent article by Richard L. Stieg, a medical doctor and researcher, titled "Roadblocks to Effective Pain Treatment" posted on April 3, 2001, at www.painconnection.org, for the National Pain Foundation. The article discusses aspects of the issue in a manner that is clear, concise, and well documented. The National Pain Foundation is recognized by the American Academy of Pain Medicine and draws on only peer-reviewed educational materials.

15. The American Academy of Pain Management should not be confused with the American Academy of Pain Medicine, abbreviated as AAPM and defined as both "the physician's voice in pain medicine," and "a medical specialty society."

16. See the NFTP's "mission statement" article citing research from the middle to late 1990s, available for review at www.paincare.org/about/mission/background.html. The article notes, "according to DEA testimony, in 1995 and 1996, 900 physicians were prose-

cuted and lost their narcotics licenses for attempting to treat
chronic pain with appropriate narcotics."

17. http://www.stoppain.org/multimedia/backpain_script.html. This
    information and much more about lower back pain, other specific
    kinds of pain, pain in general, and resources for further research
    and help is provided by the Department of Pain Medicine and
    Palliative Care, Beth Israel Hospital in New York. They have
    developed this resource center with financial support from the
    Mayday Fund, named for the French m'aidez, "help me!" and the
    birthday of its inspiration—Shirley Steinman Katzenbach. The
    Fund defines its mission to be "dedicated to alleviating the inci-
    dence, degree and consequence of human physical pain."

18. From a McGill media release April 29, 2002; http://www.mcgill.
    ca/releases/2002/april/bushnell/ (accessed August 2003). Source:
    Gaia Remerowski, McGill Office for Chemistry and Society.

19. Nessa Coyle, "Suffering in the First Person: Glimpses of Suffering
    through Patients' and Family Narratives," in *Suffering*, ed. Betty
    Ferrell (Sudbury, Mass.: Jones & Bartlett, 1995), 29–64.

20. Henry Beecher found that as many as 75 percent of the WWII
    soldiers that he studied reported needing no medication within an
    hour of significant injury ("Pain in Men Wounded in Battle,"
    Bulletin of the U.S. Army Medical Department 5 [April 1946]). By con-
    trast, a study of people with chronic back pain showed that 75
    percent had no evidence of physical injury. See John D. Loeser,
    "Low Back Pain," in *Pain*, ed. John J. Bonica, vol. 58 of *Research
    Publications: Association for Research in Nervous and Mental Disease*
    (New York: Raven Press, 1980), 363–77.

21. Elaine Scarry, *The Body in Pain: The Making and Unmaking of the
    World* (New York: Oxford University Press, 1985), 54.

22. Marni Jackson, *Pain: The Fifth Vital Sign* (New York: Crown,
    2002), 34–36.

23. This is David Morris's terminology (*Culture of Pain*).

24. Daniel Carr, "Pain Control: The New 'Whys' and 'Hows'," *Pain:
    Clinical Updates* 1 (May 1993); http://www.iasp-pain.org/PCU93a.
    html (accessed July 2003).

25. Personal communication, August, 2004.

26. Jackson, *Pain*, 178.

27. Morris, *Culture of Pain*, 9.

28. Melzack and Wall, *Challenge of Pain*.

29. Ephrem Fernandez, *Anxiety, Depression, and Anger in Pain* (Dallas:
    Advanced Psychological Resources, 2002).

30. Naomi Eisenberger, Matthew D. Lieberman, and Kipling D. Williams, "Does Rejection Hurt? An fMRI Study of Social Exclusion," *Science* 302 (2003): 290–92. Her work was preceded by others who studied a similar phenomenon in non-human subjects. For example, about twenty-five years earlier, Jaak Panksepp found in animals that "the same neurochemicals that regulate physical pain also control the psychological pain of social loss" (Jaak Panksepp, "Feeling the Pain of Social Loss," *Science* 302 [2003]: 237–39). Panksepp cites Panksepp, et al., *Neuroscience Biobehavior Revue* 4 (1980), 473 and Panksepp, in *Progress and Theory in Psychopharmacology*, ed. S. J. Cooper (London: Academic, 1981), 149–75.

31. John E. Sarno, *Mind over Back Pain: A Radically New Approach to the Diagnosis and Treatment of Back Pain* (New York: Berkley Books, 1999), 15.

32. I am grateful to Dr. Hoffman for generously sharing with me his experiences with and insights about Dr. Sarno's theory and method of treating back pain.

33. http://www.stoppain.org/education_research/glossary.html.

34. http://www.iasp-pain.org/terms-p.html.

35. http://www.theacpa.org/pain_fact_sheet.asp.

36. These terms are drawn from the IASP Task Force on Taxonomy (*Classification of Chronic Pain*, ed. H. Merskey and N. Bogduk, 2d ed. [Seattle: IASP Press, 1994], 209–14).

37. See http://www.iasp-pain.org/terms-p.html.

38. Anthony K. P. Jones, "Pain, Its Perception, and Pain Imaging," *IASP Newsletter* (May/June 1997).

39. Fernandez, *Anxiety*.

40. Karen J. Berkley, "Sexual Difference and Pain: A Constructive Issue for the Millenium," *Gender and Pain: Scientific Abstracts* (April 1998), a publication of the National Institutes of Health.

41. Melzack and Wall, *Challenge of Pain*, 71.

42. Morris, *Culture of Pain*, 246.

43. Three recently published books illustrate and describe rich understandings and interpretations of pain in cultural and historical contexts different from ours. In *The Suffering Self*, Judith Perkins tells of the revolutionary nature of early Christian attitudes toward pain in the Greco-Roman world. "By rejecting that they experienced pain or defeat, Christians rejected the power structures surrounding them, and rejected the social order they supported" (*The Suffering Self: Pain and Narrative Representation in the*

Early Christian Era [London: Routledge, 1995], 117). Ariel Glucklich sympathetically inquires about the role that pain has played in the religious experience, namely why and how people would choose to hurt themselves in the name of religion (*Sacred Pain: Hurting the Body for the Sake of the Soul* [Oxford: Oxford University Press, 2001]). I have mentioned David Morris's book above as a keen assessment, illustrated and described through literature, of the role that culture plays in making meaning out of and so providing some relief from pain.

44. I am grateful to those physicians associated with Virginia Commonwealth University's medical center who shared their experiences of and ideas for working with patients in pain and from whom I learned that a regimen of anti-depressant medication has become a regular part of treatment for such patients.

45. Arthur Frank, *The Wounded Storyteller* (Chicago: University of Chicago Press, 1995).

46. Scarry, *Body in Pain*, 5.

47. Melzack and Wall, *Challenge of Pain*, 60.

48. Scarry, *Body in Pain*, 4.

49. http://www.iasp-pain.org/terms-p.html.

50. Turk, "Assess the Person."

51. Alison McCook, "Brain Study Shows Some Feel More Pain Than Others," *Reuters Health*, E-Line, June 23, 2003.

52. Morris, *Culture of Pain*, 2.

53. Morris, *Culture of Pain*, 3.

54. Jackson, *Pain*, 349.

Notes to Chapter 2

1. David L. Kahn and Richard H. Steeves, "An Understanding of Suffering Grounded in Clinical Practice and Research," in *Suffering*, ed. Ferrell, 8–9.

2. Morris, *Culture of Pain*, 5.

3. Jack Spiro, rabbi emeritus and director of Virginia Commonwealth University's Center for Judaic Studies, delivered a lecture concerning the meaning of life at the end of which he drew listeners to think instead about meaning *in* life. The distinction that I draw here is informed by Dr. Spiro's memorable lecture.

4. Victor E. Frankl, *Man's Search for Meaning: An Introduction to Logotherapy*, part 1, trans. Ilse Lasch (New York: Pocket Books, 1963), 154, 178. The book was first published in 1959.

5. Arthur Kleinman, "'Everything That Really Matters': Social Suffering, Subjectivity, and the Remaking of Human Experience in a Disordering World," *HTR* 90 (1997): 315–35, 318.

6. Frank, *Wounded Storyteller*, 22.

7. Kleinman, "'Everything That Really Matters,'" 320.

8. That why questions have such twofold implications, pathological and cosmic, drives Margaret Mohrmann's practical inquiry into how medical personnel may recognize and handle such questions from their patients. See Mohrmann, "Someone Is Always Playing Job" in *Pain Seeking Understanding: Suffering, Medicine and Faith*. ed. Margaret E. Mohrmann and Mark J. Hanson (Cleveland: Pilgrim Press, 1999), 3.

9. He develops and explains this idea in *The Problem of Pain*, which Lewis resisted publishing under his true name on account of its problematic thesis (C. S. Lewis, *The Problem of Pain* [San Francisco: HarperSanFrancisco, 1940; repr. New York: Harper-Collins, 2001]). One wonders if his conclusions would be different if he had written this book two decades later, after watching his wife die. The narrative of Lewis's meditations on his painful loss and the process of coping with it are recorded in *A Grief Observed* (Greenwich: Seabury Press, 1961).

10. In considering "traditional theodicies," Margaret Mohrmann notes how Augustine's interpretation of pain not only conforms to this idea of pain as the deserved punishment from God but also supposes that all pain is necessarily so because of his conviction that everyone is implicated by the "original sin" of Adam and Eve. Consequently, according to Augustine's reasoning, "each human being is so tainted with the universal human choice of evil as to be guilty and deserving of whatever pain evil can inflict" (Mohrmann, *Introduction to Pain Seeking Understanding*, 3).

11. Steven Brena, *Pain and Religion: A Psychophysiological Study* (Springfield: Charles C. Thomas, 1972), 144.

12. Quoted by Mohrmann, *Introduction to Pain Seeking Understanding*, 3.

13. Betty Rolling Ferrell, "Humanizing the Experience of Pain and Illness," in *Suffering*, ed. Ferrell, 216.

14. Paul Brand and Philip Yancey, "And God Created Pain," *Christianity Today* 38 (January 10, 1994): 18–23. The article is adapted from the book.

15. Ralph Waldo Emerson, "The Tragic," in *The Complete Works of Ralph Waldo Emerson*, 12 vols. (Boston: Centenary, 1903–1904), 4:515–21.

16. Robert Smith, "Theological Perspectives" in *Suffering*, ed. Ferrell, 168–69.

17. Emmanuel Levinas, "Useless Suffering," in *The Problem of Evil*, ed. M. Larrimore (Malden, Mass.: Blackwell, 2001), 373.

18. Levinas, "Useless Suffering," 374.

19. Frankl, *Man's Search for Meaning*, 178–79.

20. Frederick W. Schmidt, Jr. *When Suffering Persists* (Harrisburg: Morehouse Publishing, 2001).

21. Anatole Broyard, *Intoxicated by My Illness, and Other Writings on Life and Death*, ed. Alexandra Broyard (New York: Clarkson Potter, 1992), 65.

22. Fyodor Dostoevsky, *The Brothers Karamazov*, trans. Constance Garnett (Garden City: Nelson Doubleday, n.d.), 219.

23. Dostoevsky, *Brothers Karamazov*, 225–26.

24. See Andrew Sung Park, *The Wounded Heart of God: The Asian Concept of Han and the Christian Doctrine of Sin* (Nashville: Abington, 1993).

25. Having noted the problems with many common interpretations, Schmidt privileges such candor and posits that such a "theology of candor" is finally the best (maybe only) appropriate response in the face of great suffering. (*When Suffering Persists*).

26. Kushner, *When Bad Things Happen*, 88.

27. William J. O'Malley, "Making Sense of Suffering and Death," in *America* 174 (1996): 96–101.

Notes to Chapter 3

1. In his preface to *Heal Thyself*, a book concerned with the reduction of Christianity to little more than a tool for health and longevity, Stanley Hauerwas distinguishes the God of worship from the god to whom we often pray when sick, a god he identifies as an idol (Joel James Shuman and Keith G. Meador, *Heal Thyself: Spirituality, Medicine, and the Distortion of Christianity* [Oxford: Oxford University Press, 2003]).

2. Morris, *Culture of Pain*, 1.

3. Claus Westermann, *The Living Psalms*, trans. J. R. Porter (Grand Rapids, Eerdmans, 1989), 75.

4. Eisenberger et al., "Does Rejection Hurt?, An fMRI Study of Social Exclusion," 290–91.

5. Arthur Frank foregrounds this observation that "bodies need voices" in his book, *The Wounded Storyteller*.

6. Jerome F. D. Creach, *Yahweh as Refuge and the Editing of the Hebrew Psalter*, JSOTSup 217 (Sheffield: Sheffield Academic Press, 1996).

7. William P. Brown, *Seeing the Psalms: A Theology of Metaphor* (Louisville: Westminster John Knox, 2002).

Notes to Chapter 4

1. William F. May, *The Patient's Ordeal*, Medical Ethics Series (Bloomington: Indiana University Press, 1994), 9, 7.

2. This is the terminology that Arthur W. Frank uses in his book, *The Wounded Storyteller*.

3. I am indebted to Frederick Schmidt for the idea of "trying on" interpretations, thereby naming the dynamic process of meaning-making that suffering elicits. Dr. Schmidt is an Episcopal priest and Director of Spiritual Life and Formation at Perkins School of Theology, Southern Methodist University, in Dallas, Texas. He has authored many books, including *When Suffering Persists*, in which he develops the argument for a new theology. He calls it a "theology of candor" that accounts for the developmental nature of interpretation in reaction to the failure of popular explanations that offer little or no comfort.

4. Schmidt, *When Suffering Persists*, 39–60.

5. Mary-Jo DelVecchio Good, et al., eds. *Pain as Human Experience: An Anthropological Perspective* (Berkeley: University of California Press, 1992), 5.

6. This primary publication by Eisenberger, et al. elicited popular attention in national newspapers as substantiation that "heartbreak's ache is real" (*Associated Press* article by Paul Recer).

7. Linda C. Garro, "Chronic Illness and the Construction of Narratives," in *Pain as Human Experience*, ed. DelVecchio, et al., 100–37.

8. Garro, "Chronic Illness," 128.

9. Kushner observes, "The Bible [. . .] repeatedly speaks of God as the special protector of the poor, the widow, and the orphan, without raising the question of how it happened that they became poor, widowed, or orphaned in the first place" (*When Bad Things Happen to Good People*, 45).

10. One way contemporary readers have sought to make sense of them is by considering the enemies to be non-human, destructive forces. In some cases, the psalms allow such interpretation, but not in every case. In what follows, I address those texts that have to do with human enemies.

11. Lawrence Kushner and David Mamet, *Five Cities of Refuge* (New York: Schocken Books, 2003), 40.
12. Park, *Wounded Heart of God.* Park is professor of theology at the United Theological Seminary.
13. I allow that justice can be perverted into a willful excuse for violence. However, the danger of such mususe should not preclude enacting justice. Reading Psalm 69 in the shadow of Good Friday, Walter Brueggemann notes, "This is not venom. [. . .] It is simply an affirmation and an insistence that evil has its own painful reward that cannot be avoided" (*The Threat of Life: Sermons on Pain, Power, and Weakness*, ed. Charles L. Campbell [Minneapolis: Fortress, 1996], 106).
14. To return to such texts in the psalms, themselves, I am indebted to Walter Brueggemann's thoughts on the matter as articulated in *Praying the Psalms* (Winona, Minn.: Saint Mary's Press, 1982).
15. Anatole Broyard, *Intoxicated by My Illness: And Other Writings on Life and Death*, ed. Alexandra Broyard [New York: Clarkson N. Potter, 1992), 25. Frank cites this as an example of the "productive desire," that can lead to service (Frank, *The Wounded Storyteller*, 39).
16. Arthur Frank notes this ideal characteristic of what he calls the "dyadic body," a profile partly dependent on Albert Schweitzer's description of the role and responsibility of members in the "community of pain" (Frank, *The Wounded Storyteller*, 40).
17. Garro, "Chronic Illness," 130.
18. Garro, "Chronic Illness," 129.
19. Schmidt, *When Suffering Persists*, 81.
20. Emmanuel Levinas, *The Levinas Reader*, ed. Sean Hand, various translators (Cambridge, Mass.: Basil Blackwell, 1989), 247.
21. *Transforming Suffering: Reflections on Finding Peace in Troubled Times by His Holiness the Dalai Lama, His Holiness Pope John Paul II, Thomas Keating, Thubten Chodron, Joseph Goldstein, and Others*, ed. Donald W. Mitchell and James Wiseman (New York: Doubleday, 2003), 16.
22. *The Levinas Reader*, trans. Richard Cohen, 44.
23. *The Levinas Reader*, trans. Richard Cohen, 46.
24. Kushner and Mamet, *Five Cities of Refuge*, 6.
25. This is also the conclusion that Schmidt draws in his book *When Suffering Persists*.
26. Schmidt, *When Suffering Persists*, 101.

Notes to Chapter 5

1. This is the terminology that Walter Brueggemann uses to denote

strict principles of justice according to commonly agreed upon laws and regulations. Infractions, in such a system, are met with specific punishments. Walter Brueggemann, "A Shape for Old Testament Theology: 1, Structure Legitimation: 2, Embrace of Pain," *CBQ* 47 (1985): 28–46.

2. Benjamin R. Foster, *From Distant Days: Myths, Tales, and Poetry of Ancient Mesopotamia* (Bethesda, Md.: CDL Press, 1995), 412.

3. Augustine, *City of God*, XIV, 14–15. Augustine was the bishop of Hippo from 396–430 CE.

4. Blaise Pascal, *Minor Works*. trans. O. W. Wright, Harvard Classics, ed. Charles W. Eliot (New York: P. F. Collier & Son, 1910), 48:373.

5. Caton also wrote the book *What a Blessing She Had Chloroform: The Medical and Social Response to the Pain of Childbirth from 1800 to the Present* (New Haven: Yale University Press, 1999). His 30-minute lecture is available on the internet at http://www.medinfo.ufl.edu/other/histmed/caton/index.html.

6. Indeed, at the risk of stating the obvious, it may be instructive to remember that the psalms, with other ancient writings and traditions that I have cited here, derive from a period preceding anesthesia. Caton attributes C. S. Lewis with the observation that great religions such as Judaism and Christianity got their start in, and so their writings reflect, a period before anesthesia. Much, then, that informed their theologies were efforts to come to terms with such difficult human experiences as unrelieved illness and pain.

7. Arthur Kleinman, "Pain and Resistance" in *Pain as Human Experience: An Anthropological Perspective*, ed. Mary-Jo DelVecchio Good, et al. (Berkeley: University of California Press, 1992), 175.

8. Kleinman, "Pain and Resistance," 178.

9. Kleinman, "Pain and Resistance," 180.

10. Robert Smith, "Theological Perspectives," in *Suffering*, ed. Ferrell, 165.

11. Kleinman, "Pain and Resistance," 181.

12. Kleinman, "Pain and Resistance," 177.

13. Kleinman, "Pain and Resistance," 179.

14. Kleinman, "Pain and Resistance," 181.

15. Kleinman, "Pain and Resistance," 177.

16. Kleinman, "Pain and Resistance," 176–77.

17. Kleinman, "Pain and Resistance," 171.

18. This expression comes from Kleinman, "'Everything That Really Matters,'" 315–35.

19. Smith, "Theological Perspectives," in *Suffering*, ed. Ferrell, 164–65.

20. Not only can such an interpretation be destructive of the patient, but Patrick Coyne, R. N. and M. S. N., observes that it is also painfully destructive to his or her family. In his work administering palliative care to patients, most of whom are in the end stages of cancer, Coyne has seen the devastating effects that a person's interpretation of their pain as punishment has on the people who love him or her. Coyne speaks with great sadness of lost opportunities for connection with family and friends because of interpreting pain as a necessary penalty and because this image of great suffering is the last (and frequently most powerful) one that such family and friends have of the dying patient (personal communication, August 2004).

21. Kleinman, "'Everything That Really Matters,'" 317.

22. Kleinman, "'Everything That Really Matters,'" 318.

23. Kleinman, "'Everything That Really Matters,'" 320.

24. Kleinman, "'Everything That Really Matters,'" 318. In making this observation, Kleinman draws on the work of the anthropologist Veena Das.

25. Susan Sontag, *Illness as Metaphor and AIDS and Its Metaphors* (New York: Anchor Books, 1990), 3. *Illness as Metaphor* was originally published in 1978 and *AIDS and Its Metaphors* in 1989.

26. This description by biblical scholar and professor Tod Linafelt of the book of Lamentations articulates a distinction poignantly evident also in Psalm 38. *Surviving Lamentations: Catastrophe, Lament, and Protest in the Afterlife of a Biblical Book* (Chicago: Chicago University Press, 2000), 17.

Notes to Chapter 6

1. This is the first line of a poem by Emily Dickinson. (*The Complete Poems of Emily Dickinson*. ed. Thomas H. Johnson [Boston: Little, Brown, 1957]).

2. Frank, *The Wounded Storyteller*, 97, 99.

3. Jackson, *Pain*, 145.

4. Dickinson, *Complete Poems*, 323–24.

5. Frank, *The Wounded Storyteller*, 110.

6. Frank, *The Wounded Storyteller*, 101.

7. Gerald G. May, *The Dark Night of the Soul: A Psychiatrist Explores the*

Connection Between Darkness and Spiritual Growth (San Francisco: HarperSanFrancisco, 2004), 42.

8. Dickinson, *Complete Poems*, 47.

9. Broyard, *Intoxicated by My Illness*, 30.

10. Garrett Keizer, *The Enigma of Anger: Essays on a Sometimes Deadly Sin* (San Francisco: Jossey-Bass, 2002), 222.

11. Matthew 12:10-13; Mark 3:1-5; Luke 6:6-10.

12. Keizer, *Engima of Anger*, 241.

13. We see such theology articulated clearly in Isaiah 45:6-7, both the uniqueness of God and consequently the attribution to God of light and darkness, peace, and evil; so too Deuteronomy 32:39.

14. Elliot N. Dorff, "Rabbi, Why Does God Make Me Suffer?" in *Pain Seeking Understanding*, ed. Mohrmann and Hanson, 119.

15. Keizer, *Enigma of Anger*, 268.

16. The spelling of this word makes it possible to read as a noun of place/location or as a prepositional phrase. That is, the *mem* may be either a preformative, indicating a place; or a preposition, translated "from" or "from within." (Paul Joüon, *A Grammar of Biblical Hebrew*, trans. and rev. T. Muraoka, 2 vols.[Rome: Editrice Pontificio Istituto Biblico, 1996], 1:255–60). Its vocalization suggests that it should be read as a noun of place.

17. Jackson, *Pain*, 144.

18. Carole Fontaine, "Arrows of the Almighty," in *ATR* 66 (1984): 244.

19. May, *Dark Night of the Soul*, 72.

20. John of the Cross, *Dark Night of the Soul*, trans. and ed. E. Allison Peers; 3d ed. (Garden City, NY: Image Books, 1959), ch. 16, parag. 11.

21. Mary C. Earle, *Broken Body, Healing Spirit: Lectio Divina and Living with Illness* (Harrisburg: Morehouse, 2003), 72.

22. May contemplates this aspect of the saints' desire for God in *Dark Night of the Soul*, 54–57.

23. May, *Dark Night of the Soul*, 74.

24. May, *Dark Night of the Soul*, 197.

25. Keizer, *Enigma of Anger*, 16.

26. Remen, *My Grandfather's Blessings*, 104–5.

Notes to Chapter 7

1. John S. Lunn, "Spiritual Care in a Multi-Religious Context," in *Journal of Pain and Palliative Care Pharmacotherapy* 17 (2003): 156.

2. The second half of the psalm is so different from the first that many scholars conclude that they were originally two separate

psalms. Whatever the case, these parts compose one psalm now, and together they are thought-provoking and insightful.

3. Joseph Campbell, *Hero with a Thousand Faces* (1949; repr., Cleveland: World Publishing, 1970), 108.

4. Campbell, *Hero*, 109.

5. Campbell, *Hero*, 150–51.

6. Campbell, *Hero*, 190.

7. Campbell, *Hero*, 157–58.

8. Campbell, *Hero*, 162.

9. Personal conversation, July 2004.

10. Sontag, *Illness as Metaphor*, 3.

11. Oliver Sacks, *A Leg to Stand On* (New York: Summit Books, 1984), 111.

12. Kat Duff, *The Alchemy of Illness* (New York: Pantheon Books, 1993), xii.

13. Underscoring the psalmist's sense of alienation, the Hebrew suggestively toggles back and forth between genders. That is, the bicolon reads, "I am a worm (feminine noun), not a man (masculine noun that usually refers specifically to male people), a joke (feminine noun) of a human being (masculine noun that may be used of a male person or more generally of people), and despised (masculine participle) by people (a term used generally of people)." One may surmise that the sufferer's gender or sexual orientation is in question; however, this is not made explicit in the psalm and so remains conjecture.

14. May, *Patient's Ordeal*, 15.

15. May, *Patient's Ordeal*, 35.

16. May, *Patient's Ordeal*, 142.

17. Thomas G. Couser, *Recovering Bodies: Illness, Disability, and Lifewriting*, Wisconsin Studies in American Autobiography (Madison: University of Wisconsin Press, 1997).

18. Keizer, *Enigma of Anger*, 257.

19. This was composed by freelance writer Eric Minton.

20. Couser, *Recovering Bodies*, 180.

21. May, *Patient's Ordeal*, 20–24.

22. Duff, *Alchemy of Illness*, 81.

23. Cliff Edwards discesses this letter in *The Shoes of Van Gogh: A Spiritual and Artistic Journey to the Ordinary* (New York: Crossroad, 2004), 20.

24. Frank, *The Wounded Storyteller*, 119.

25. Duff, *Alchemy of Illness*, 132.

26. This phrase concludes Mary Oliver's poem, "Wild Geese."

27. Frank, *The Wounded Storyteller*, 127–28.

28. Cliff Edwards introduced me to the quiet power of Vincent Van Gogh's *Pear Tree in Bloom with Butterfly* that forms the backdrop of this book's cover. One bare and broken branch, a butterfly barely visible yet present, and spindly branches exploding in bursts of bloom make it seem a fitting image for this book.

29. Vincent Van Gogh, *The Complete Letters of Vincent Van Gogh*, 2d ed., 3 vols. (Boston: New York Graphic Society, 1978), 1:206.

30. Cliff Edwards, *Van Gogh and God: A Creative Spiritual Quest* (Chicago: Loyola University Press, 1989), 79.

31. Margaret E. Mohrmann, *Medicine as Ministry: Reflections on Suffering, Ethics, and Hope* (Cleveland: Pilgrim Press, 1995), 42.

32. Duff, *Alchemy of Illness*, 146.

Notes to Chapter 8

1. Margaret Morganroth Gullette, "Ordinary Pain," *North American Review* 278, no. 3 (1993): 41–46.

2. Gullette, "Ordinary Pain," 46.

3. Susan Greenhalgh, *Under the Medical Gaze: Facts and Fictions of Chronic Pain* (Berkeley: University of California Press, 2001).

4. Sarno, *Mind over Back Pain*, 31.

5. Sarno, *Mind over Back Pain*, 82.

6. This is the title of Larry Bouchard's chapter in the book, *Pain Seeking Understanding*, ed. Mohrmann and Hanson.

7. Although Psalm 6 came to be included in the Middle Ages among the collection of "Penitential Pss," its lack of confession is unique and so has raised questions about identifying it with the other six Penitential Psalms (32, 38, 51, 102, 130, 143).

8. The psalm returns in verse 4 to a request for God to help. It is subtly different from that which opened the psalm, however, insofar as it does not imply sinfulness. Instead, the psalmist pleads that YHWH "return," "draw out," and "deliver." Each of these terms merits brief discussion. Although the term translated "return" could be understood as the action of desisting from punishing judgment, it may simply be, here, a request for attention. Indeed, this verb frequently connotes coming back. Here, it is as though God had abandoned the psalmist who, in reaction, pleads for God's presence. The psalmist follows this plea with another. In the second, the psalmist chooses a Hebrew term that evokes an image of God's deliverance involving "drawing out/off," perhaps pulling

the psalmist along and thereby extending and/or saving his or her life. The third request, defined by a verb meaning "to save, deliver" again reflects an earnest desire that YHWH attend to the psalmist's condition. That the verb can mean not simply "to save" but also "to deliver" suggests that the psalmist wants God actively to position the psalmist in a new way for a new purpose. That is, while the psalmist clearly expresses a desire to live and not die, it may be that with this term she also tells of wanting a life with direction and purpose.

9. Larry D. Bouchard, "Holding Fragments," in *Pain Seeking Understanding*, ed. Mohrmann and Hanson, 26.

10. Bouchard, "Holding Fragments," 22.

11. Bouchard, "Holding Fragments," 22.

12. Mohrmann, "Someone is Always Playing Job," in *Pain Seeking Understanding*, ed. Mohrmann and Hanson, 78.

13. Peter C. Craigie raises this third possibility in his commentary (*Psalms 1–50*, Word Biblical Commentary 19 [Waco, Tex.: Word Books, 1983], 92).

14. The brief sentence is identical to Baruch's lament in Jeremiah 45:3. However, to Baruch God responds immediately, though not with comfort or encouragement. God's response to Baruch in the book of Jeremiah is rather an oracle of yet more destruction and fierce purpose for the man as an individual.

15. In the context of this observation, Mohrmann notes that those in pain include the family of a patient as well as the suffering patient himself or herself (personal communication, June 2004).

16. Duff, *Alchemy of Illness*, xi.

17. Gullette, "Ordinary Pain," 41.

18. Sarno, *Mind over Back Pain*, 85.

19. Sarno, *Mind over Back Pain*, 81.

20. Although verse 7 shares with verse 6 the tone of grief, it also represents the beginning of a move into action. The psalmist declares that she is angry/annoyed/vexed.

21. Gullette, "Ordinary Pain," 43.

22. Gullette, "Ordinary Pain," 45.

23. Jackson, *Pain*, 99.

24. The Hebrew term that I translate "those holding me back," usually refers to human enemies; but it is also sometimes used of general distress (e.g., Deuteronomy 4:30). Although the word that I translate "those who make" is commonly used of people and of God, it is not exclusively so (e.g., its subject is a wild ass in Job 24:5).

25. E.g. "Hot-Headed Approach to Heart Disease," *Harvard Heart Letter* (May 2004).

26. A recent study by Patricia Eng, ScD, of the Harvard School for Public Health demonstrates how the expression of anger may improve a person's health. See "Expressing Anger May Protect against Stroke, Heart Disease," in *Heart Disease Weekly* (March 2, 2003), 6.

27. Keizer, *Enigma of Anger*, 10.

28. Keizer, *Enigma of Anger*, 358.

29. Keizer, *Enigma of Anger*, 10.

30. Bouchard, "Holding Fragments," 21.

31. Dorothee Soelle, *Suffering*, trans. Everett R. Kalin (Philadelphia: Fortress, 1975).

32. Soelle, *Suffering*, 73.

33. Albert H. Keller, "When Truth is Mediated by a Life," in *Pain Seeking Understanding*, ed. Mohrmann and Hanson, 50.

Notes to Chapter 9

1. Wendell Berry, *Another Turn of the Crank* (Washington, D.C.: Counterpoint, 1995), 105.

2. I use the term *modern* here to refer simply to the literature of our time, without distinguishing it by specific dates or from literature labeled "postmodern."

3. I use *dying* here to refer to that condition wherein there is no cure, no turning back from the path leading to death; time is notably limited although the duration may vary.

4. Garrison Keillor, "In Autumn We All Get Older Again," *Time* 146.19 (November 6, 1995): 90.

5. Keillor, "In Autumn," 90.

6. For insightful reflection on and elegant explanation of this aspect of the matter of theodicy, I am indebted to the work of Daniel P. Sulmasy, "Finitude, Freedom, and Suffering," in *Pain Seeking Understanding*, ed. Mohrmann and Hanson, 83–102.

7. This Hebrew word means both "heart" and "mind."

8. Sulmasy, "Finitude, Freedom, and Suffering," in *Pain Seeking Understanding*, ed. Mohrmann and Hanson, 96.

9. Sherwin Nuland, *How We Die: Reflections on Life's Final Chapter* (New York: Alfred A. Knopf, 1994), 43.

10. Nuland, *How We Die*, 43.

11. Personal communication, July 2004.

12. Stephen Levine, *Who Dies?: An Investigation of Conscious Living and Conscious Dying* (Garden City, N.Y.: Anchor Books, 1982), 115.

13. Jackson, *Pain*, 357.

14. The words that I have translated "ones dying" are from a word that can mean "belonging to the group of" plus a noun for death. The same string of words appears in Psalm 79, which can be said to express a communal experience similar to the individual's in Psalm 102.

15. Levine, *Who Dies?* 117.

16. Levine, *Who Dies?* 124.

17. Ernest J. Gaines, *A Lesson before Dying* (New York: Vintage Books, 1993), 234.

18. Levine, *Who Dies?* 16.

19. Rabbi emeritus and director of Virginia Commonwealth University's Center for Judaic Studies, Dr. Jack Spiro, brought my attention to this collection of sayings that circulated on the internet.

20. Nuland, *How We Die*, xvii.

21. Kleinman, "'Everything That Really Matters,'" 332.

22. Washington Matthews, *Navaho Legends*, Memoirs of the American Folk-Lore Society 5 (1897), 77–78.

23. Garrison Keillor, "Crankiness in Decline, Says Old Guy: Youth-obsessed America Has Made it Tough to Age with Crabby, Righteous Anger," *Time* 160.8 (August 19, 2002): 172.

24. Nuland, *How We Die*, 86.

25. Nuland, *How We Die*, 87.

26. Sulmasy, "Finitude, Freedom, and Suffering, " in *Pain Seeking Understanding*, ed. Mohrmann and Hanson, 101.

27. May, *Patient's Ordeal*, 153–54.

28. Nuland, *How We Die*, 268.

29. Jackson, *Pain*, 314.

30. Kleinman, "'Everything That Really Matters'," 330.

31. Berry, "Health is Membership," 102.

Notes to the Conclusion

1. Remen, *My Grandfather's Blessings*, 139.

Works Cited

Allen, Leslie C. "The Value of Rhetorical Criticism in Psalm 69." *Journal of Biblical Literature* 105 (1986): 577–82.

Allmark, Peter. "Death with Dignity." *Journal of Medical Ethics* 28 (2002): 255–57.

Anderson, Bernhard, with Steven Bishop. *Out of the Depths: The Psalms Speak for Us Today*. 3rd ed. Louisville: Westminster John Knox, 2000.

Attig, Thomas. *How We Grieve: Relearning the World*. New York: Oxford University Press, 1996.

Avalos, Hector. *Illness and Health Care in the Ancient Near East: The Role of the Temple in Greece, Mesopotamia, and Israel*. Harvard Semitic Museum Monographs 54. Atlanta: Scholars Press, 1995.

Bakan, David. *Disease, Pain, Sacrifice: Toward a Psychology of Suffering*. Chicago: University of Chicago Press, 1968.

Barbour, John D. "The Bios of Bioethics and the Bios of Autobiography." In *Caring Well: Religion, Narrative, and Health Care Ethics*. Edited by D. H. Smith, 43–63. Louisville: Westminster John Knox, 2000.

Bates, Maryann S. *Biocultural Dimensions of Chronic Pain: Implications for Treatment of Multi-ethnic Populations*. SUNY Series in Medical Anthropology. Albany: State University of New York Press, 1996.

Beecher, Henry K. "Pain in Men Wounded in Battle." *The Bulletin of the U.S. Army Medical Department* 5 (April 1946).

Berger, Peter L. *The Sacred Canopy: Elements of A Sociological Theory of Religion*. New York: Doubleday, 1967.

Berkley, Karen J. "Sexual Difference and Pain: A Constructive Issue for the Millennium." *Gender and Pain: Scientific Abstracts* (April 1998).

Berquist, Jon L. *Controlling Corporeality: The Body and the Household in Ancient Israel*. New Brunswick, NJ: Rutgers University Press, 2002.

Berry, Wendell. *Another Turn of the Crank*. Washington, DC: Counterpoint, 1995.

Birkeland, Harris. *'Ani und 'Anaw in den Psalmen*. Translated by E. L. Rapp. Oslo: I Kommisjon Hos Jacob Dybwad, 1933.

Bouchard, Larry D. "Holding Fragments." In *Pain Seeking Understanding*. Edited by Margaret E. Mohrmann and Mark J. Hanson, 13–28. Cleveland: Pilgrim Press, 1999.

Brand, Paul, and Philip Yancey. *Pain: The Gift Nobody Wants*. New York: HarperCollins, 1993.

— — —. "And God Created Pain." *Christianity Today* 38 (1994): 18–23.

Brena, Steven. *Pain and Religion: A Psychophysiological Study*. Springfield: Charles C. Thomas, 1972.

Broyard, Anatole. *Intoxicated by My Illness, and Other Writings on Life and Death*. Edited by Alexandra Broyard. New York: Clarkson Potter, 1992.

Brown, William P. *Seeing the Psalms: A Theology of Metaphor*. Louisville: Westminster John Knox Press, 2002.

Brueggemann, Walter. *Praying the Psalms*. Winona, Minn.: Saint Mary's Press, 1982.

— — —. "A Shape for Old Testament Theology: 1, Structure Legitimation; 2, Embrace of Pain." *Catholic Biblical Quarterly* 47 (1985): 28–46.

— — —. "A Gospel Language of Pain and Possibility." *Horizons in Biblical Theology* 13 (1991): 95–133.

— — —. *The Threat of Life: Sermons on Pain, Power, and Weakness*. Edited by Charles L. Campbell. Minneapolis: Fortress, 1997.

Bushnell, Catherine. "Picturing Your Pain." McGill Office for Chemistry and Society. McGill media release April 29, 2002. http://www.mcgill.ca/releases/2002/april/bushnell/ (accessed August, 2003).

Campbell, Joseph. *Hero with a Thousand Faces*. 1949. Reprint, Cleveland: World Publishing, 1970.

Carr, Daniel. "Pain Control: The New 'Whys' and 'Hows'." *Pain: Clinical Updates* 1 (May 1993). http://www.iasp-pain.org/ PCU93.htm (accessed July 2003).

Caton, Donald. "History of Medicine." http://www.medinfo.ufl.edu/ other/histmed/caton/index.html (accessed June 2004).

Charlton, James I. *Nothing About Us Without Us: Disability Oppression and Empowerment*. Berkeley: University of California Press, 1998.

Clark, David. "'Total Pain,' Disciplinary Power and the Body in the Work of Cicely Saunders, 1958–1967." *Social Science & Medicine* 49 (1999): 727–36.

Cohen, Darlene. *Turning Suffering Inside out: a Zen Approach to Living with Physical and Emotional Pain*. Boston, Mass.: Shambhala, 2002.

Couser, G. Thomas. *Recovering Bodies: Illness, Disability, and Life-writing*. Madison: University of Wisconsin Press, 1997.

Coyle, Nessa. "Suffering in the First Person: Glimpses of Suffering through Patients' and Family Narratives." In *Suffering*. Edited by Betty Rolling Ferrell, 29–64. Sudbury, Mass.: Jones & Bartlett, 1995.

Craigie, Peter C. *Psalms 1–50*. Word Biblical Commentary 19. Waco: Word Books, 1983.

Creach, Jerome F. D. *Yahweh as Refuge and the Editing of the Hebrew Psalter*. JSOTSup 217. Sheffield: Sheffield Academic Press, 1996.

Dallek, Robert. "The Medical Ordeals of JFK." *Atlantic Monthly* 290 (December 2002): 49–52, 54f.

Davis, Bryn D. *Caring for People in Pain*. New York: Routledge, 2000.

DeAngelis, Catherine D. "Pain Management." *Journal of the American Medical Association* 290 (2003): 2480–81.

DelVecchio Good, Mary-Jo, Paul E. Brodwin, Byron J. Good, and Arthur Kleinman, eds. *Pain as Human Experience: An Anthropological Perspective*. Berkeley: University of California Press, 1992.

Dennis, Geoffrey and Jackie Herzlinger. "The Congregational Nurse, A New Ally toward Making the Synagogue a Center of Healing." *Central Conference of American Rabbis Journal* (2003): 67–74.

Dickinson, Emily. *The Complete Poems of Emily Dickinson*. Edited by Thomas H. Johnson. Boston: Little, Brown, 1957.

Dorff, Elliot N. "Rabbi, Why Does God Make Me Suffer?" In *Pain Seeking Understanding*. Edited by Mohrmann and Hanson, 115–25. Cleveland: Pilgrim Press, 1999.

Doestoevsky, Fyodor. *The Brothers Karamazov*. Translated by Constance Garnett. Garden City, N.Y.: Nelson Doubleday, n.d.

Duff, Kat. *The Alchemy of Illness*. New York: Pantheon Books, 1993.

Dunson, Miriam. *A Very Present Help: Psalm Studies for Older Adults*. Louisville: Geneva Press, 1999.

Earle, Mary C. *Broken Body, Healing Spirit: Lectio Divina and Living with Illness*. Harrisburg: Morehouse, 2003.

Edwards, Cliff. *Van Gogh and God: A Creative Spiritual Quest*. Chicago: Loyola University Press, 1989.

— — —. *The Shoes of Van Gogh: A Spiritual and Artistic Journey to the Ordinary*. New York: Crossroad, 2004.

Eisenberger, Naomi I., Matthew D. Lieberman, and Kipling D. Williams. "Does Rejection Hurt? An fMRI Study of Social Exclusion." *Science* 302 (2003): 290–92.

Emerson, Ralph Waldo. "The Tragic." In *The Complete Works of Ralph Waldo Emerson*. 12 vols. Boston: Centenary, 1903–1904. 4:515–21.

Eng, Patricia. "Expressing Anger May Protect against Stroke, Heart Disease." *Heart Disease Weekly* (March 2, 2003): 6.

Ersek, Mary, and Betty R. Ferrell. "Providing Relief for Cancer Pain by Assisting in the Search for Meaning." *Journal of Palliative Care* 10 (1994): 19–22.

Fernandez, Ephrem. *Anxiety, Depression, and Anger in Pain*. Dallas: Advanced Psychological Resources, 2002.

Ferrell, Betty Rolling. "Humanizing the Experience of Pain and Illness." In *Suffering*. Edited by Ferrell, 210–16. Sudbury, Mass.: Jones & Bartlett, 1995.

Fichter, Joseph H. *Religion and Pain: The Spiritual Dimensions of Health Care*. New York: Crossroad, 1981.

Fontaine, Carole. "Arrows of the Almighty." *Anglican Theological Review* 66 (1984): 243–48.

"Former HHS Secretary Sullivan, Former Sugeron General Satcher Announce Educational Tool to Fight 'Epidemic' of Untreated Pain." *US Newswire* via COMTEX, September 8, 2003.

Foster, Benjamin R. *From Distant Days: Myths, Tales, and Poetry of Ancient Mesopotamia*. Bethseda, Md.: CDL Press, 1995.

Frank, Arthur. *The Wounded Storyteller*. Chicago: University of Chicago Press, 1995.

Frankl, Viktor E. *Man's Search for Meaning: An Introduction to Logotherapy.* Translated by Ilse Lasch, with preface by Gordon W. Allport. Rev. and enl. ed. New York: Pocket Books, 1963.

Gaines, Ernest J. *A Lesson Before Dying.* New York: Vintage Books, 1993.

Garro, Linda C. "Chronic Illness and the Construction of Narratives." In *Pain as Human Experience.* Edited by DelVecchio Good, et al., 100–37. Berkeley: University of California Press, 1992.

Gerstenberger, Erhard S. *Psalms, Part 2, and Lamentations.* Forms of the Old Testament Literature 15. Grand Rapids: Eerdmans, 2001.

Glucklich, Ariel. "Sacred Pain and the Phenomenal Self." *Harvard Theological Review* 91 (1998): 389–412.

— — —. *Sacred Pain: Hurting the Body for the Sake of the Soul.* Oxford: Oxford University Press, 2001.

Greenhalgh, Susan. *Under the Medical Gaze: Facts and Fictions of Chronic Pain.* Berkeley: University of California Press, 2001.

Groopman, Jerome. "God at the Bedside." *New England Journal of Medicine* 350 (2004): 1176–78.

Gullette, Margaret Morganroth. "Ordinary Pain." *North American Review* 278 (1993): 41–46.

Hardcastle, Valerie Gray. *The Myth of Pain: Philosophical Psychopathology.* Cambridge, Mass.: MIT Press, 1999.

Harmon, Louise. *Fragments on the Deathwatch.* Boston: Beacon Press, 1998.

Hawthorn, Jan, and Kathy Redmond. *Pain: Causes and Management.* Malden, Mass.: Blackwell Science, 1998.

Holewa, Kathryn A., and John P. Higgins. "Palliative Care—The Empowering Alternative: A Roman Catholic Perspective." *Trinity Journal* 24 (2003): 207–19.

Holladay, William L. *The Psalms Through Three Thousand Years: Prayerbook of a Cloud of Witnesses.* Minneapolis: Fortress, 1993.

"Hot-Headed Approach to Heart Disease." *Harvard Heart Letter,* 2004.

Hull, John M. *In the Beginning There Was Darkness: A Blind Person's Conversations with the Bible.* Harrisburg: Trinity Press International, 2001.

IASP Task Force on Taxonomy. *Classification of Chronic Pain.* Edited by H. Merskey and N. Bogduk, 209–14. Seattle: IASP Press, 1994.

Jackson, Marni. *Pain: The Fifth Vital Sign.* New York: Crown , 2002.

Jaki, Stanley L. *Praying the Psalms: A Commentary.* Grand Rapids: Eerdmans, 2001.

John of the Cross. *Dark Night of the Soul.* 3rd ed. Translated and edited by E. Allison Peers. Garden City, N.Y.: Image Books, 1959.

Jones, Anthony K. P. "Pain, Its Perception, and Pain Imaging." *International Association for the Study of Pain Newsletter*, 1997.

Joüon, Paul. *A Grammar of Biblical Hebrew.* Translated and revised by T. Muraoka. 2 vols. Rome: Editrice Pontificio Instituto Biblico, 1996.

Kahlo, Frida. *The Diary of Frida Kahlo: An Intimate Self-Portrait.* Introduction by Carlos Fuentes. Essay and Commentaries by Sarah M. Lowe. La Vaca Independiente S.A. de C.V., Mexico: Harry N. Abrams, 1995.

Kahn, David L., and Richard H. Steeves. "An Understanding of Suffering Grounded in Clinical Practice and Research." In *Suffering.* Edited by Ferrell, 13–28. Sudbury, Mass.: Jones & Bartlett, 1995.

Keillor, Garrison. "In Autumn We All Get Older Again." *Time* 146.19 (November, 6 1995): 90.

— — —. "Crankiness in Decline, Says Old Guy: Youth-obsessed America Has Made it Tough to Age with Crabby, Righteous Anger." *Time* 160.8 (August 19, 2002): 72.

Keizer, Garret. *The Enigma of Anger: Essays on a Sometimes Deadly Sin.* San Francisco: Jossey-Bass, 2002.

Keller, Albert H. "When Truth is Mediated by a Life." In *Pain Seeking Understanding.* Edited by Mohrmann and Hanson, 50–61. Cleveland: Pilgrim Press, 1999.

Kleinman, Arthur. "Pain and Resistance." In *Pain as Human Experience.* Edited by DelVecchio Good, et al., 169–97. Berkeley: University of California Pres, 1992.

— — —. "'Everything That Really Matters': Social Suffering, Subjectivity, and the Remaking of Human Experience in a Disordering World." *Harvard Theological Review* 90 (1997): 315–35.

Kushner, Harold S. *When Bad Things Happen to Good People.* New York: Schocken Books, 1981. Reprint, New York: Avon Books, 1983.

Kushner, Lawrence, and David Mamet. *Five Cities of Refuge.* New York: Schocken Books, 2003.

Levinas, Emmanuel. *The Levinas Reader*. Edited by Sean Hand. Various Translators. Cambridge, Mass.: Basil Blackwell, 1989.

— — —. "Useless Suffering." In *The Problem of Evil*. Edited by M. Larrimore, 371–80. Malden, Mass.: Blackwell, 2001.

Levine, Stephen. *Who Dies?: An Investigation of Conscious Living and Conscious Dying*. Garden City, N.Y.: Anchor Books, 1982.

Lewis, C. S. *The Problem of Pain*. San Francisco: HarperSanFrancisco, 1940. Reprint. New York: HarperCollins, 2001.

— — —. *A Grief Observed*. Greenwich: Seabury Press, 1961.

Limburg, James. *Psalms for Sojourners*. Rev. ed. Minneapolis: Fortress , 2002.

Linafelt, Tod. *Surviving Lamentations: Catastrophe, Lament, and Protest in the Afterlife of a Biblical Book*. Chicago: Chicago University Press, 2000.

Loeser, John. D. "Low Back Pain." In *Pain*. Edited by John J. Bonica, 363–77. Research Publications: Association for Research in Nervous and Mental Disease. New York: Raven Press, 1980.

Lunn, John S. "Spiritual Care in a Multi-Religious Context." *Journal of Pain and Palliative Care Pharmacotherapy* 17 (2003): 153–66.

Matthews, Washington. *Navaho Legends*. Memoirs of the American Folk-Lore Society 5 (1897).

May, Gerald G. *Dark Night of the Soul: A Psychiatrist Explores the Connection Between Darkness and Spiritual Growth*. San Francisco: HarperSanFrancisco, 2004.

May, William F. *The Patient's Ordeal*. Medical Ethics Series. Bloomington: Indiana University Press, 1994.

— — —. *The Physician's Covenant: Images of the Healer in Medical Ethics*. Rev. ed. Louisville: Westminster John Knox , 2000.

McCaffery, Margo. *Pain: Clinical Manual*. St. Louis: Mosby, 1999.

McCook, Alison. "Brain Study Shows Some Feel More Pain Than Others." *Reuters Health E-Line* (June 23, 2003): n.p.

McCutchan, Stephen P. "Framing Our Pain: The Psalms in Worship." *Christian Ministry* 26 (1995): 18–20.

Meldrum, Marcia L. "Capsule History of Pain Management." *Journal of the American Medical Association* 290 (2003): 2470–75.

Melzack, Ronald, and Patrick D. Wall. *The Challenge of Pain*. New York: Penguin, 1982. Reprint of *The Puzzle of Pain*. New York: Penguin Education, 1973.

Menn, Esther. "No Ordinary Lament: Relecture and the Identity of the Distressed in Psalm 22." *Harvard Theological Review* 93 (2000): 301–42.

Miller, Andrew. *Ingenious Pain*. San Diego: Harcourt Brace, 1997.

Miller, Patrick D., Jr. *Interpreting the Psalms*. Philadelphia: Fortress, 1986.

Mitchell, Donald W., and James Wiseman, eds. *Transforming Suffering: Reflections on Finding Peace in Troubled Times by His Holiness the Dalai Lama, His Holiness Pope John Paul II, Thomas Keating, Thubten Chodron, Joseph Goldstein, and Others*. New York: Doubleday, 2003.

Mohrmann, Margaret E. *Medicine as Ministry: Reflections on Suffering, Ethics, and Hope*. Cleveland: Pilgrim Press, 1995.

———. "Someone is Always Playing Job." In *Pain Seeking Understanding*. Edited by Mohrmann and Hanson, 62–79. Cleveland: Pilgrim Press, 1999.

Morris, David B. *The Culture of Pain*. Berkeley: University of California Press, 1993.

Naegele, Kaspar D. *Health and Healing*. Edited by Elaine Cumming. San Francisco: Jossey-Bass, 1970.

Nuland, Sherwin. *How We Die: Reflections on Life's Final Chapter*. New York: Alfred A. Knopf, 1994.

Oates, Wayne E. and Charles E. *People in Pain: Guidelines for Pastoral Care*. Philadelphia: Westminster Press, 1985.

O'Malley, William J. "Making Sense of Suffering and Death." *America* 174 (1996): 96–101.

Owens, Dorothy M. *Hospitality to Strangers: Empathy and the Physician-Patient Relationship*. AAR Academy Series 100. Atlanta: Scholars Press, 1999.

Panksepp, Jaak. "Feeling the Pain of Social Loss." *Science* 302 (2003): 237–39.

Park, Andrew Sung. *The Wounded Heart of God: The Asian Concept of Han and the Christian Doctrine of Sin*. Nashville: Abingdon, 1993.

Pascal, Blaise. *Minor Works*. Edited by Charles W. Eliot. Translated by O. W. Wright. New York: P. F. Collier & Son, 1910.

Penchansky, David. *What Rough Beast? Images of God in the Hebrew Bible*. Louisville: Westminster John Knox, 1999.

Perkins, Judith. *The Suffering Self: Pain and Narrative Representation in the Early Christian Era*. London: Routledge, 1995.

Permut, Joanna Baume. *Embracing the Wolf: A Lupus Victim and Her Family Learn to Live with Chronic Disease*. Atlanta: Cherokee, 1989.

Petrie, Asenath. *Individuality in Pain and Suffering*. Rev. ed. Chicago: Chicago University Press, 1978.

Remen, Naomi Rachel. *Kitch Table Wisdom: Stories that Heal*. New York: Riverhead Books, 1996.

———. *My Granfather's Blessings: Stories of Strength, Refuge, and Belonging*. New York: Reiverhead Books, 2000.

Renner, Johannes, T. E. "Aspects of Pain and Suffering in the Old Testament." *Colloquium* 15 (1982): 32–42.

Robinson, Rebecca L., Howard G. Birnbaum, Melissa A. Morley, Tamar Sisitsky, Paul E. Greenberg, and Ami J. Claxton. "Economic Cost and Epidemiological Characteristics of Patients with Fibronyalia Claims." *Journal of Rheumatology* 30 (2003): 1318–25.

Roy, Ranjan. *Social Relations and Chronic Pain*. Plenum Series in Rehabilitation and Health. New York: Kluwer Academic, 2002.

Sacks, Oliver. *A Leg to Stand On*. New York: Summit Books, 1984.

Sanford, John A. *Healing and Wholeness*. New York: Paulist Press, 1977.

Sanford, Matthew. *Waking: A Passage into Body*. Emmaus, Penn.: Rodale, forthcoming.

Sarna, Nahum M. *Songs of the Heart: An Introduction to the Book of Psalms*. New York: Schocken Books, 1993.

Sarno, John E. *Mind over Back Pain: A Radically New Approach to the Diagnosis and Treatment of Back Pain*. Rev. ed. New York: Berkeley Books, 1999.

Scarry, Elaine. *The Body in Pain: The Making and Unmaking of the World*. New York: Oxford University Press, 1985.

Schmidt, Frederick W., Jr. *When Suffering Persists*. Harrisburg: Morehouse , 2001.

Schweizer, Harold. *Suffering and the Remedy of Art*. Albany: State University of New York Press, 1997.

Shuman, Joel James. *The Body of Compassion: Ethics, Medicine, and the Church*. Radical Traditions Series. Boulder: Westview, 1999.

Shuman, Joel James, and Keith G. Meador. *Heal Thyself: Spirituality, Medicine, and the Distortion of Christianity*. Oxford: Oxford University Press, 2003.

Smith, David H, ed. *Caring Well: Religion, Narrative, and Health Care Ethics*. Louisville: Westminster John Knox, 2000.

Smith, Robert. "Theological Perspectives." In *Suffering*. Edited by Ferrell, 159–72. Sudbury, Mass.: Jones & Bartlett, 1995.

Smolkin, Mitchell T. *Understanding Pain: Interpretation and Philosophy*. Malabar, Fla.: Robert E. Krieger, 1989.

Soelle, Dorothee. *Suffering*. Translated by Everett R. Kalin. Philadelphia: Fortress, 1975.

Sontag, Susan. *Illness as Metaphor and AIDS and Its Metaphors*. New York: Anchor Books, 1990.

Stewart, Walter F., Judith A. Ricci, Elsbeth Chee, David Morganstein, and Richard Lipton. "Lost Productive Time and Cost Due to Common Pain Conditions in the US Workforce." *JAMA* 290 (2003) 2443–54.

Stull, Bradford T. *Religious Dialectics of Pain and Imagination*. SUNY Series in Rhetoric and Theology. Albany: State University of New York, 1994.

Sulmasy, Daniel P. "Finitude, Freedom, and Suffering." In *Pain Seeking Understanding*. Edited by Mohrmann and Hanson, 83–102.

Sylva, Dennis. *Psalms and the Transformation of Stress: Poetic-Communal Interpretation and the Family*. Louvain Theological and Pastoral Monographs 16. Louvain: Peeters , 1993.

Tambasco, Anthony J., ed. *The Bible on Suffering: Social and Political Implications*. New York: Paulist, 2001.

Taylor, Barbara Brown. "The Day We Were Left Behind." In *The Best Spiritual Writing, 1999*. Edited by Phillip Zaleski, 258–65. San Francisco: Harper Collins, 1999.

Terrien, Samuel L. *The Psalms: Strophic Structure and Theological Commentary*. Grand Rapids: Eerdmans, 2003.

Turk, Dennis C. "Assess the Person, Not Just the Pain." *Pain: Clinical Updates* 1 (September 1993): n.p. http://www.iasp-pain.org/PCU93c.html. Accessed July 19, 2003.

Van Gogh, Vincent. *The Complete Letters of Vincent Van Gogh*. 2d ed. 3 vols. Boston: New York Graphic Society, 1978.

Weiner, Kathryn. "Pain is an Epidemic." *AAPM Special Message*, 2002.

Westermann, Claus. *The Psalms: Structure, Content and Message.* Translated by Ralph D. Gehrke. Minneapolis: Augsburg, 1980.

— — —. *The Living Psalms.* Translated by J. R. Porter. Grand Rapids: Eerdmans, 1989.

Zborowski, Mark. *People in Pain.* San Francisco: Jossey-Bass, 1960.

Index